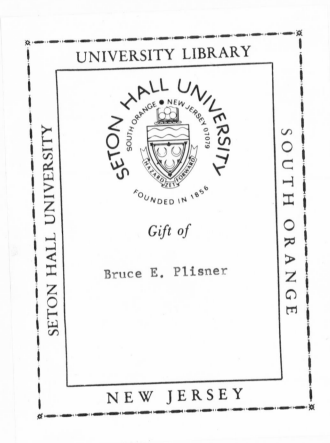

MANAGEMENT OF THE POISONED PATIENT

Based upon papers presented at the Joint Symposium of the American Academy of Clinical Toxicology, the American Association of Poison Control Centers, and the Canadian Academy of Clinical Toxicology.

Edited by

Barry H. Rumack, M.D.

and

Anthony R. Temple, M.D.

Published by

SCIENCE PRESS

Princeton

PROGRAM COMMITTEE
FOR THE SYMPOSIUM

Barry H. Rumack, M.D.
General Chairman

Griffith E. Quinby, M.D., M.P.H.
American Academy of Clinical Toxicology

William O. Robertson
American Association of Poison Control Centers

Yves LaCasse, M.D.
Canadian Academy of Clinical Toxicology

Library of Congress Cataloging in Publication Data

Main entry under title:

Management of the poisoned patient.

    1. Toxicology—Congresses. 2. Medical emergencies—Congresses. I. Rumack, Barry H. II. Temple, Anthony R. III. American Academy of Clinical Toxicology. IV. American Association of Poison Control Centers. V. Canadian Academy of Clinical Toxicology.

RA1191.M36   615.9'08   77-78689
ISBN 0-89500-026-1

Printed in the United States of America

CONTENTS

FOREWORD

While the beginnings of Clinical Toxicology may be dated back to the time of Socrates or before, few advances have been made until the past twenty years. Interest was spurred during the mid nineteen fifties with the institution of the Poison Control Center System and the formation of the American Association of Poison Control Centers shortly afterward. The AAPCC met in conjunction with the Pediatric Academy because the major interest of the Poison Control effort was toward children.

In the late nineteen sixties, the American Academy of Clinical Toxicology was formed with the intent of creating a scientific forum for the advancement of clinical toxicology. This group existed to encourage competence among those who would view this field as a primary interest. Toward this end a board was created to examine this field and ensure continued education and training.

More recently, the Canadian Academy of Clinical and Analytical Toxicology was formed to deal with those problems unique to that country and provide a strong voice in this medical specialty.

In August of 1976, these three organizations held their annual convention together for the first time. This joint meeting brought together a wide variety of people interested in all aspects of clinical toxicology. The results of many of the symposia held during the joint meeting have been brought together in published form for the first time, in this book. Many of the ideas presented here are new and unique contributions to the medical literature, and provide valuable information useful to those working in the field of clinical toxicology and medical management of both human and animal poison cases.

The book is divided essentially into two parts. The first part consists of sixteen major papers presented at the joint symposia. The latter part of the book presents eight short papers which, while they are relatively brief, are included because of their topical importance.

It is hoped that the results of the 1977 joint meeting to be held in Quebec will be as successful as this first meeting, and provide further contributions of current research, methodology, and applications for the use of those working in the field.

BARRY H. RUMACK, M.D.
ANTHONY R. TEMPLE, M.D.
Editors

PERIPHERAL NEUROPATHY DUE TO METHYL n-BUTYL KETONE AND RELATED SOLVENTS

James M. Parker, M.D.
Assistant Professor, Division of Neurology, Department of Medicine, The Ohio State University Hospitals, Columbus, Ohio

J. Norman Allen, M.D.
Professor of Neurology and Director, Division of Neurology, Department of Medicine, The Ohio State University Hospitals, Columbus, Ohio

Jerry R. Mendell, M.D.
Associate Professor, Division of Neurology, Department of Medicine, The Ohio State University Hospitals, Columbus, Ohio

ABSTRACT

An industrial outbreak in 1973 resulted in 86 cases of a sensorimotor polyneuropathy of distinctive pattern. Deficits on physical examination and EMG were distal in distribution and appeared to affect large myelinated fibers. Weakness was generally limited to muscles of forearms and hands and lower legs and feet with minimal atrophy. Sensory loss principally involved pinprick, temperature and touch deficits over hands and feet. Onset was insidious and delayed progression of the disorder after elimination of toxic exposure was often observed. Attack rates were related to intensity of solvent exposure, to the time of introduction of MBK and to hours of work. Clinical cases were not found in a similar plant in which MBK was not employed. Cessation of new case development and recovery of original cases occurred after removal of MBK and simultaneous environmental improvement. Isolated cases of similar pattern were reported elsewhere after exposure to MBK. Experimentally, continuous exposure to MBK at

*200-600 ppm resulted in clinical neuropathy in chickens
at 4-5 weeks, cats at 5-8 weeks, and rats at 11-12 weeks.
Earliest evidence of histological abnormalities were detected in rats at 4 weeks after exposure to 150 ppm. A
synergistic effect was found with methyl-ethyl ketone,
since exposure of rats to 150 ppm MBK and 1,500 ppm MEK
yielded histological neuropathy by 11 days. Morpholog-
ical findings were distinctive, with focal axonal swelling, myelin denudation, accumulation of dense masses of
neurofilaments, normal numbers of neurotubules, and delayed axoplasmic flow rates. Biopsy of a human case
exposed to MBK but also to lead showed a similar patho-
logical process. An identical neuropathy can be seen
with n-hexane exposure, and the two solvents may yield
a common ultimate toxin.*

In 1973 an outbreak of a previously unknown peripheral
neuropathy occurred in Columbus, Ohio (1). In June 1973
a patient hospitalized on the Neurosurgery Service at
The Ohio State University Hospitals was diagnosed as
having a peripheral neuropathy felt to be toxic in nature. He provided a list of six of his co-workers with
similar symptoms. Peripheral neuropathy was subsequently diagnosed in all of them.

They were employed at a coated fabrics plant which
manufactured wall coverings and other materials with
extensive use of dyes and solvents during the process.
A survey of the plant then began involving neurological,
electrodiagnostic and clinical chemistry evaluations.
All employees having abnormal electrodiagnostic studies
received detailed neurologic examinations. One thousand
and fifty-seven employees were studied of whom eighty-
six were found to have unexplained peripheral neuropathy,
most quite mild. The clinical pattern was one of motor,
sensory and sometimes both motor and sensory involvement. The onset of motor symptoms was gradual with
painless weakness beginning distally in feet and hands.
Atrophy was occasionally seen as well as weight loss

and muscle cramps (2).

The sensory pattern was characterized by paresthesias and numbness in the distal extremities with maximal decrease in pinprick, touch and temperature with variable and rather slight loss of vibration. Position sense was relatively preserved. Loss of tendon reflexes was minimal and confined to distal reflexes such as finger and ankle jerks. Cranial nerve involvement as well as autonomic defects and diffuse reflex loss were absent. Electromyographic abnormalities consisted of signs of denervation, including positive waves, fibrillations, fasciculations and abnormal motor unit action potentials which were maximal distally and decreased proximally. In affected cases nerve conduction velocities were moderately reduced, ranging from 25 to 45 m/sec. Normal peroneal conduction velocity (mean) is 50 m/sec (3).

Laboratory values were generally normal. Occasional elevations in liver enzymes were seen but without a consistent pattern (2). CSF was normal except for elevated protein present in one out of four samples examined. A number of employees had decreased erythrocyte acetylcholinesterase values and increased serum butyrylcholinesterase--this did not, however, correlate with neuropathy (3). A number of patients showed progression up to several months after cessation of exposure.

As the clinical evaluation of the employees began so did the search for the causative agent. The possibility of relationship of the neuropathy to known etiologies was entertained but the clinical pattern differed from many known toxins such as lead, arsenic, thallium, acrylamide and carbon disulfide. A resemblance was noted to the neuropathy of n-hexane and remotely to tri-ortho-cresyl phosphate. These agents were either absent from the plant or present only in trace amounts (1).

In order to more easily apply epidemiological methods

a scoring system was devised. Scores were obtained by
assigning weighted numerical values to electrodiagnostic
and neurologic abnormalities (3). A relationship had
been discovered between the neuropathy and certain areas
of the plant, especially those involved with the printing operations with their use of dyes and solvents (1).

Prior to the outbreak a change in solvents had occurred.
The previous solvents, primarily methyl ethyl ketone
(MEK) and to a lesser extent methyl isobutyl ketone
(MIBK) had been used for some years but because of MIBK's
photo conversion and higher volatility, methyl n-butyl
ketone (MBK) was introduced and gradually substituted
during summer and fall of 1972 (1). The onset of cases
occurred as this process reached its peak. The cases
occurred largely in those having the highest exposure
to MBK in the print department, the print operators,
their helpers and those who cleaned the dye pans. There
was no correlation of the age of those workers ill or
not ill in the print department (1). The duration of
symptoms of all employees with peripheral neuropathy
tended to be less than one year. Non-print department
employees had a lower incidence of unexplained neuropathy but a variety of neurologic diseases was found.

Atmospheric sampling for MEK and MBK revealed highest
concentrations in the area of the print machines--up to
516 ppm of MEK and 36 ppm for MBK (1). Investigation
was carried out in a California plant using a similar
printing process but where MBK had never been used. No
neuropathy was found.

Based upon these findings MBK was presumptively identified as the toxic agent. MBK was eliminated from the
plant along with concomitant improvements in ventilation
and work procedures (1). These changes occurred as the
investigation was underway. The neuropathies gradually
improved and no new cases appeared. The patient with
the most severe involvement continues to show a mild
neuropathy but has returned to work.

Factors supporting the identification of MBK as the causative agent include the onset of the neuropathy correlating with exposure to MBK with none occurring prior to its use. Also, there was no relationship of presence or severity of neuropathy to number of years in the plant, indicating no influence of previous agents. Since improvement in ventilation was brought about simultaneously with removal of MBK it is conceivable that an undetected or unknown agent could have contributed but it would have had to have exposure and concentration characteristics identical to MBK.

Other cases of neuropathy following exposure to MBK have been reported in spray painters and others using it as a solvent (4). A peripheral nerve biopsy in one of these cases revealed pathologic changes identical to those found in animals (5). Chickens, cats, rats, and mice were exposed to both MBK and MEK in an environmental chamber (6). Clinical signs of neuropathy developed in chickens after 4 weeks at 200 ppm, in cats after 5-8 weeks at 400 ppm, and in rats after 12 weeks at 400 ppm. No clinical signs were observed in mice although histopathologic changes were present. Exposure of all these animals to MEK at 1500 ppm resulted in no clinical signs of neuropathy. Histopathologic findings in these animals included focal axonal swellings which were found to consist of densely packed masses of neurofilaments (6, 7). Neurotubules were unchanged. Internodal and paranodal myelin loss was also found. Because an interaction of MBK and MEK was considered possible, rats were exposed to both MBK and MEK simultaneously which resulted in the histologic changes occurring after shorter exposure times and to a greater degree than with MBK alone (5).

A relationship has been proposed between MBK neuropathy and that of n-hexane (8). The clinical picture is similar and the histopathology is virtually identical. There may be an ultimate toxin common to both. Bacteria can metabolize n-hexane to MBK, and one of the metabolites of MBK, 2-5 hexandione has been shown to produce an experimental neuropathy identical to MBK (9). MBK has been found in the urine of patients with hyperglycinemia (10) and methyl malonic aciduria (11) although neuropathy is not a feature of these conditions.

In summary, a toxic neuropathy diagnosed in workers at a coated fabrics plant in Columbus, Ohio in 1973 was determined, after clinical and epidemiologic studies and animal experiments, to be due to exposure to the industrial solvent methyl n-butyl ketone.

REFERENCES

1. Billmaier D, Yee H, Allen N, et al: Peripheral neuropathy in a coated fabrics plant. *J Occup Med* October 1974

2. Allen N, Mendell J, Billmaier D, et al: An outbreak of a previously undescribed toxic poly- neuropathy due to industrial solvent. *Trans Am Neurol Assn* 99:23-28, 1974.

3. Allen N, Mendell J, Billmaier D, et al: Toxic polyneuropathy due to methyl n-butyl ketone. *Arch Neurol* 32:209, April 1975.

4. Mallov J: MBK neoropathy among spray painters. *JAMA* 235:1455, 1976.

5. Mendell J, Saida K, Ganasia M, et al: Toxic poly- neuropathy produced by methyl n-butyl ketone. *Science* 185:787-789, August 1974.

6. Saida K, Mendell J, Weiss H: Peripheral nerve changes induced by methyl n-butyl ketone and potentiated by methyl ethyl ketone. *J Neuropathol and Exp Neurol* 35:207-225, 1976.

7. Spencer P, Schaumberg H, Raleigh R, et al: Nervous system degeneration produced by the industrial solvent methyl n-butyl ketone. *Arch Neurol* 32:219-222, April 1975.

8. Means E, Prockop L, Hooper G: Pathology of lacquer thinner induced neuropathy. *Ann Clin Lab Sci* 6:240-250, 1976.

9. Spencer P, Schaumberg H: Experimental neuropathy produced by 2.5 hexandione: A major metabolite of the neurotoxic industrial solvent methyl n-butyl ketone. *J. Neurol Neurosurg Psychiat* 38:771-775, 1975.

8

10. Menkes J: Idiopathic hyperglycinemia: Isolation and identification of three previously undescribed urinary ketones. *J Pediat* 69:113-421, 1966.

11. Rosenberg L, Lilljequist A, Hsia Y: Methylmalonic aciduria. *New Eng J Med* 278:1319-1322.

NEUROPSYCHOLOGICAL DEFICITS OF CHRONIC INHALANT ABUSERS*

G. James Berry, M.D.
Director, Addiction Research Unit, Division of
Psychiatric Services, Denver Department of Health and
Hospitals, Denver, Colorado

Robert K. Heaton, Ph.D.
Assistant Professor of Clinical Psychology, University
of Colorado Medical Center, Denver, Colorado

Michael W. Kirby, Ph.D.
Assistant Clinical Professor of Psychology, University
of Colorado Medical Center, Denver, Colorado

ABSTRACT

A group of 75 youths with extensive histories of solvent inhalation were evaluated neuropsychologically in
an attempt to determine whether solvent abuse is associated with cerebral dysfunction. They were compared
to a group of control subjects matched for age, sex,
ethnicity, educational and socio-economic background.

Although solvents have been previously associated
with peripheral neurotoxicity, there has been a pau-
city of information concerning their effects on central
nervous system functions. Data are presented on the
neuropsychological functioning, intelligence, and personality profiles of this group of solvent abusers.

---

*This work was supported by H.E.W. Grant No. 1 H81
DA 01687 from the National Institute on Drug Abuse.

INTRODUCTION

It is not precisely known just how dangerous the practice of voluntary solvent inhalation is in terms of the central nervous system. An evaluation of the literature on potential toxicity is difficult and does not lead to many definite conclusions. Many of the available reports are based on industrial exposures, anesthetic exposures, or animal experiments; and to what extent these data are applicable to the recreational user, or abuser of solvents is unknown.

There has been considerable concern about the toxic potential of solvents for brain tissues; however there are remarkably few reports relative to the inhalant abuse situation concerning either acute or chronic effects. Certainly volatile solvents are capable of producing peripheral neurotoxicity (1, 2, 3, 4, 5, 6, 7, 8); and several authors suggest inhalation of solvents is capable of causing permanent brain damage in humans (1, 9, 10, 11, 12), but the evidence for chronic central nervous system toxicity remains fragmentary. The few additional reports which do exist are often contradictory, with some investigators finding their chronic solvent users impaired, while others report normal neuropsychological functioning (13, 14, 15, 16, 17, 18).

The present study was undertaken in an attempt to develop information concerning the neuropsychological functioning of a group of chronic users of volatile solvents. Standardized procedures which yield quantitative results were used to investigate a variety of personality, intelligence, and neuropsychological factors. Similar data have been collected from non-using control subjects. Data from the experimental and control groups were compared in an effort to determine if chronic inhalation of volatile solvents is associated with deficits in neuropsychological functioning. This study is still in progress, and data reported from this initial group of subjects should be considered preliminary.

METHOD

Subjects:

Our interest in assessing inhalant users neuropsychologically was stimulated initially by the previous experience of one of the authors who encountered a group
of inhalant abusing youths referred to a drug abuse
treatment program under his direction. These youths
were subsequently recruited as subjects for the present
study. They also provided access to other inhalant
abusers and to non-using peers, who served as experimental and control subjects respectively. Excluded from
the study were those individuals whose primary language
was other than English, those with a Full Scale I.Q. of
less than 80, those with histories of psychiatric hos-
pitalizations, periods of unconsciousness exceeding 10
minutes, seizure disorders, or other medical conditions
which would be expected to influence the test results.
Also excluded were individuals with histories of significant use of other drugs, including alcohol. Neuropsychological testing was not conducted, or the data
were deleted, if a subject's self-report, clinical examination, or urine toxicology screen indicated the use
of any psychotropic substance in the preceding 72 hours.

Experimental group:

The experimental group consisted of 37 chronic in-
halers of volatile substances, who conformed to the
exclusion criteria. They had been inhaling solvents
an average of 5.5 years (range 1.5 to 17 years), with
some beginning as early as age 6 or 7 years. Subjects
had experienced an average of more than 7,400 voluntary
exposures to solvents, sniffing an average 3.7 times
each day. The preferred substances in the Denver area
are the metallic paints, followed closely by clear
paints and varnishes for those individuals who make
some attempt to conceal their use of inhalants.

The average age at the time of testing was 18.3 years
(range 15 to 29), with males outnumbering females 33

to 4. Twenty-seven percent of the sample were Anglo,
62% were Mexican American, and 11% American Indian.
We have found no Black users in our experience, and the
reason remains unclear to us. The subjects had been
enrolled in school 9.7 years on the average, with only
16% attending school or employed at the time of testing.
They had been arrested an average of 5 times in the
preceding 24 months and convicted 2.3 times in the same
period. Nearly a third considered their fathers to
abuse alcohol. Subjects' self-reports indicated they
had refrained from sniffing a minimum of 3 days at the
time of testing, with some abstinent as much as 1 year.

Control group:

The control group consisted of 11 subjects who were
either siblings or peers of the experimental subjects.
The two groups were comparable with respect to age, sex,
ethnicity, educational level, and socioeconomic and
cultural backgrounds. Attempts were made to control
also for the use of other substances including alcohol.
Individuals reporting any use of inhalants were excluded
from the control group (Table I).

The experimental and control groups are closely
matched on the demographic or descriptive variables
which might be presumed to have the greatest influence
on neuropsychological performance, i.e., age, sex,
ethnicity, and education. The groups were also similar
on a number of measures of socioeconomic status, self-
report of illegal activity, family characteristics
including use of drugs and alcohol, and histories of
medical conditions including head trauma.

Table II reflects some of the drug use data collected,
including the percent of subjects in each group who
indicated they had ever used a substance and the age at
first use. Any use during the 90 days prior to testing
is indicated also. Substances are listed sequentially
according to the order in which the groups began using
them. That is, alcohol was the substance first used by

each group, followed by marihuana. The solvent users began sniffing about the same time they began using marihuana. Although many individuals in both groups have experimented at least once with several classes of drugs, additional data, not present here, concerning chronicity and frequency of each substance used demonstrates their use has been infrequent with the exception of alcohol and marihuana. Where between group differences do exist, they are in a direction which we presume would favor the solvent users. That is, a greater percentage of the control group have used some substances, beginning at an earlier age, than has the experimental group (Table II).

Psychological Testing

Psychological tests were administered individually by a technician who was not informed which subjects were users and which were controls. Many of the tests make up the neuropsychological test battery developed by Halstead (19) and Reitan (20,21). The sensitivity of this battery to cerebral lesions has been validated by numerous studies over the last 20 years involving a variety of populations with documented brain lesions (22). Several other tests were included, most of which are given in conjunction with the core Halstead-Reitan Battery in many clinical settings. The complete series of tests includes measures of personality, intelligence, attention and various cognitive functions, motor proficiency, sensory-perceptual functions, aphasia and related disorders, and verbal learning and memory. The rationale and procedure for each of the 20 tests utilized in this study has been described in detail previously (19,21,23, 24,25,26,27,28,29,30,31,32), and will not be replicated here.

RESULTS

Data were analyzed by establishing frequency distributions and measures of central tendency for each demographic or descriptive variable. Additionally, the

neuropsychological data from each group were subjected
to analysis of variance. Degrees of freedom were
established using the derivation of Dixon and Massey (33)
which compensates for samples of small n, and for dis-
crepancies of sample size between groups. Differences
between group means were elevated using the t-test, and
levels of significance were established for each dependent
variable.

Table III presents the means and standard deviations
of the Minnesota Multiphasic Personality Inventory
(MMPI) scores for our two groups. The inhalant group
scored significantly higher on the F, or Validity Scale,
as well as on four of the clinical scales: Depression
(Scale 2), Psychasthenia (Scale 7), Schizophrenia
(Scale 8), and Social Introversion (Scale 0).

Their high scores on the F Scale raise some question
as to whether subjects in the inhalant group may have
made deliberate attempts to emphasize psychopathology.
This possibility cannot be ruled out, but is considered
unlikely for two reasons. First, since the test data
were being collected by an independent research team,
the subjects would have had no reason to suspect that
appearing psychiatrically disturbed would affect their
medical treatment or status with the legal authorities.
And second, a high F score would be expected and usually
would not invalidate profiles in a population of young
delinquents showing this group's mixed patterns of
antisocial and schizoid traits on their MMPI clinical
scales (34,35,36,37). (Table III)

As an aid in analyzing the MMPI clinical scale data,
Figure 1 shows the mean MMPI profiles for the two groups.
The major elevations on these profiles correspond well
with the modal profiles of each group. Thus, the most
frequent two-scale code for the group (n = 6) involve
Psychopathic Deviate (Scale 4) and Hypomania (Scale 9).
This is the classic sociopathy configuration, usually
seen with impulsive, self-centered, manipulative

individuals, who tend to abuse drugs and engage in other antisocial acting out (34,36). By contrast, the inhalant subjects' profiles tend to be more elevated in general (reflecting more serious psychopathology), and their modal two-scale code involves Scales 8 and 9 (n = 11). In addition, the inhalant profiles are similar to those of the controls in that Scale 4 is frequently elevated (among the top three clinical scales in 18), and are different in that they show significantly greater elevations of Scales 2, 7, 8, and 0.

Taken together, the MMPI results suggest that the inhalant subjects are similar to the controls in that they are self-centered, immature people with strong tendencies to undercontrol their impulses and get into trouble with their environments. However, the inhalant subjects appear to be more seriously disturbed as a group, and in particular are apt to show more general dissatisfaction with their lives, more difficulty with thinking and communication, poorer judgment, greater feelings of social alienation and distrust of others, and to be more ruminative and overideational (34,35, 36). (Fig. 1)

Table IV presents means, standard deviations, and statistically significant group differences for the intelligence test data.

Mean scaled scores on all the individual WAIS subtests are higher for the control group than for the inhalant group, but the only statistically significant difference was on Comprehension. Differences were substantial on the Verbal (9 points) and Full Scale (8 points) I.Q. values, however, both of these reaching statistical significance. Bearing in mind that the minimum I.Q. for inclusion in this study was 80, twenty-two (60 percent) of the inhalant subjects earned Full Scale I.Q.'s in Wechsler's Dull Normal range (80-89), whereas only one control subject scored this low. Subjects in both groups tended to earn their lowest

scores on the Information, Vocabulary, and Arithmetic
subtests, a finding which may reflect a combination of
marginal school adjustment and cultural deprivation
(Table IV).

Results on the neuropsychological test battery
(Tables V and VI) are similar to those seen on the
WAIS in that, even though many of the differences do
not reach statistical significance, the inhalant group's
mean scores are worse than those of the controls in
every instance. Also, almost half of the comparisons
using the individual test scores did yield statistically
significant results. These scores include the Tactual
Performance Test Time/Block and Memory scores, the
Tactile Form Recognition score, the Hand Dynamometer
and Maze Coordination scores, and both measures of
learning efficiency and the delayed memory score on
the Story Memory Test. The trend of these results is
graphically demonstrated in Figure 2, which shows the
group mean T scores computed for the WAIS I.Q. values,
the seven measures from Halstead's original neuropsychological battery, and the two neuropsychological
summary scores. Note that the inhalant group did
significantly worse than the controls on both neuropsychological summary measures. Using previously
established cutoff points (27,29) fifteen of the
inhalant subjects scored in the brain damaged range
on the Halstead Impairment Index, the Average Impairment Rating, or both. No control subject scored in
the brain damaged range on either measure (Fig. 2).

DISCUSSION

We would like to emphasize again this is a preliminary
report based upon small sample sizes. Although the
groups were closely matched and statistically significant between-group differences were obtained on a number
of measures, the size of the control group is marginal.
Several other considerations are pertinent when attempting to interpret these results.

The confounding effect of using other drugs or alcohol is a potentially serious one. The drug-use histories of the two groups were very similar in many respects, but not identical. The intriguing aspect of this is that where trends or significant differences in drug use did exist, they were in a direction which would tend to diminish the differences in neuropsychological performance of the groups. For instance, the control group used more alcohol at an earlier age. We would expect the higher use of alcohol to diminish the performance of the control group, if it had any effect. The experimental group might have appeared even more impaired had they been compared to a control group identical in their use of substances other than solvents.

Major issues raised by our neuropsychological test results concern which of the group differences were likely caused by inhalant abuse, and which may have been pre-existing or even predisposing factors to that abuse.

In the case of the personality test findings, the MMPI profiles of both groups are quite consistent with the subjects' known histories of delinquency. The more severe psychopathology and emphasis upon schizoid features and general dysphoria suggested with the inhalant group might well have been predisposing factors to the use of these substances. Their use of solvents may have helped them avoid stresses associated with peer relations and other (e.g., school and family) aspects of their lives, and also may have provided a temporary sense of well being which appears to be relatively lacking in their normal state. On the other hand, the acute (but more or less continuous) cognitive and affective changes caused by heavy use of these substances throughout their adolescent periods would be expected to adversely effect these subjects' psychosocial development. In the absence of objective data concerning the earlier psychiatric status of

these subjects, we suspect that both of the above
cause-effect relationships apply in most of these cases.
That is, while less adequate pre-exposure psychosocial
functioning may have made inhalant abuse attractive to
them, the very frequent inhalation of solvents throughout the adolescent period probably exacerbated any pre-
existing psychiatric disturbance.

Our results indicate that the inhalant abusers are
currently less adequate than the controls in terms of
both past accumulated knowledge (Verbal I.Q.) and a
variety of current adaptive abilities dependent upon
brain functions (expanded Halstead-Reitan Battery).
Moreover, previous validation research with the neuropsychological test battery employed in this study
strongly suggests an organic etiology for many of the
deficits shown by the inhalant subjects. The ability
deficits noted with our inhalant subjects are of sufficient magnitude to warrant concern and continued
research into the possibility that extensive recreational inhalation of these substances may cause irreversible effects on the central nervous system.

The implications of the psychological test results
for each subject's everyday functioning depends upon
his specific pattern of strengths and deficits. However, the prospects of many inhalant subjects for successful future social and vocational functioning appear
to be marginal. In many cases the MMPI results would
predict continuing problems in establishing and main-
taining satisfying peer relationships, poor abilities
to hold up and respond adaptively to stresses, peculiar
and at times confused and disorganized thinking, and
tendencies towards unpredictable behavior which reflects
poor judgment and forethought. As mentioned above,
ability deficits for the inhalant subjects are variable.
However, those most apt to effect everyday functioning
often include problems with new concept formation,
inefficiency in following complex sequential procedures,
marginal "common sense" in a variety of social contexts,

poor learning and memory for new verbal material,
inefficiency in psychomotor problem solving, and poor
fine motor coordination.

The preliminary data presented from our study obviously raise more questions than they answer. However,
our group of inhalant abusers performed more poorly
than the control group on such a variety of neuropsychological tests that it is difficult to escape
the conclusion the inhalant abusers are impaired.

Table I

Descriptive Characteristics

Item	Inhalant Users	S.D.	Control Group	S.D.
N	37		11	
Age	18.3	3.9	17.4	0.9
Sex (Male)	89%		91%	
Ethnicity				
Anglo	27%		27%	
Mexican American	62%		64%	
American Indian	11%		9%	
Formal Education	9.7	1.9	8.6	1.3
Attending School or Employed	16%		0%	
Arrests During Last 2 Years	5.0	5.9	4.9	4.7
Convictions During Last 2 Years	2.3	4.5	1.4	1.2
Age at First Drug Use	10.7	3.2	9.8	3.9

Table II

Drug Use Histories

	Ever Used (%)	Used in Last 90 Days (%)	Age of First Use
Alcohol			
Inhalant Users	100	14	10.7
Controls	91	64	9.8
Marihuana			
Inhalant Users	100	86	12.8
Controls	100	100	10.8
Solvents			
Inhalant Users	100	86	12.8
Controls	0	0	----
Amphetamines			
Inhalant Users	73	35	11.3
Controls	82	64	12.9
Barbiturates			
Inhalant Users	54	19	15.0
Controls	64	18	14.0
Hallucinogens			
Inhalant Users	54	16	15.8
Controls	55	18	14.6
Cocaine			
Inhalant Users	38	14	16.6
Controls	55	9	15.6
Heroin			
Inhalant Users	24	0	16.9
Controls	45	0	15.5

Table III

Minnesota Multiphasic Personality Inventory
T Scores Means, Standard Deviations, and
t Values for Inhalant and Control Groups

MMPI Scales[1]	Inhalant (Mean)	S.D.	Control (Mean)	S.D.	t
L	49.05	6.50	51.27	9.43	-0.73
F	79.68	17.80	64.45	9.56	3.70**
K	44.46	7.31	48.91	9.83	-1.39
Hypochondriasis	58.19	14.25	53.36	7.70	1.46
Depression	62.57	13.72	53.45	9.35	2.52*
Hysteria	55.40	11.59	55.36	6.09	0.01
Psychopathic Deviate	71.03	12.15	67.36	7.39	1.22
Masculinity-Femininity	57.57	10.59	56.09	8.26	0.48
Paranoia	66.86	12.89	59.64	7.75	2.29
Psychasthenia	67.84	14.54	57.91	8.75	2.78**
Schizophrenia	80.65	18.73	62.82	6.95	4.78**
Hypomania	74.73	11.63	74.36	10.65	0.09
Social Introversion	57.57	10.57	49.00	8.73	2.71*

 * p < .05
** p < .01

[1] Scores on Clinical Scales include appropriate K corrections.

Wechsler Adult Intelligence Scale

Subtest	Inhalant (Mean)	S.D.	Control (Mean)	S.D.	t
Information	6.52	2.24	6.73	2.10	-0.29
Comprehension	7.24	2.17	10.73	3.29	-3.30**
Arithmetic	7.24	2.49	8.00	2.24	-0.95
Similarities	8.59	2.97	9.64	3.10	-0.98
Digit Span	8.11	2.49	9.09	1.97	-1.36
Vocabulary	6.35	2.06	7.73	1.85	-2.11
Verbal I.Q.	88.16	9.44	96.82	9.99	-2.55*
Digit Symbol	7.95	2.54	8.36	1.69	-0.63
Picture Completion	9.32	1.97	10.09	1.51	-1.36
Block Design	9.43	2.52	10.09	2.12	-0.86
Picture Arrangement	9.27	2.04	10.09	1.87	-1.25
Object Assembly	8.70	3.05	9.82	2.56	-1.21
Performance I.Q.	93.92	11.20	99.55	8.25	-1.81
FULL SCALE I.Q.	89.97	8.97	97.73	8.26	-2.67*

* p < .05
** p < .01

Table V

Neuropsychological Test Data

Test	Inhalant Group	S.D.	Control Group	S.D.	t
Halstead Impairment Index	0.36	0.23	0.20	0.14	2.89**
Average Impairment Rating	1.29	0.37	1.01	0.31	2.47*
Cognition-Attention-Memory					
Category Test (errors)	61.08	24.97	47.18	21.68	1.80
Trail Making Test (Part A)	30.41	12.70	27.00	6.21	1.21
Trail Making Test (Part B)	94.73	42.50	75.91	28.47	1.70
Tactual Performance Test:					
Memory	8.14	1.03	8.82	0.75	-2.41*
Location	5.32	2.22	6.18	1.66	-1.38
Seashore Rhythm (correct)	24.49	4.69	26.27	6.89	-1.59
Speech Perception (errors)	7.16	5.52	5.45	1.92	1.58
Story Memory:					
Trials to criterion	2.77	1.37	1.64	0.81	3.37**
Information per trial	7.89	4.38	13.50	6.48	-2.67*
Memory	2.56	1.90	0.91	1.63	2.79*

* p < .05
** p < .01

Table VI

Neuropsychological Test Data

Test	Inhalant Group	S.D.	Control Group	S.D.	t
Language and Communications					
Aphasia (errors)	11.09	6.58	8.20	4.32	1.28
Sensory-Perceptual Functions					
Perceptual (errors)	2.00	3.72	0.36	0.67	2.53
Spatial Relations (errors)	2.39	0.90	2.18	0.40	1.06
Tactile Form Recognition (seconds)	17.66	3.27	15.36	2.12	2.74*
Motor Functions					
Finger Oscillation	93.07	10.69	96.55	5.80	-1.40
Hand Dynamometer (kilograms)	79.53	19.01	96.00	19.52	-2.47*
Grooved Pegboard (seconds)	151.19	30.58	147.73	19.68	0.44
Static Steadiness (errors)	82.28	45.79	63.91	40.65	1.23
Maze Coordination (errors)	42.00	20.99	28.45	12.17	2.53*
Tactual Performance Test:					
Total time per block	0.57	0.28	0.38	0.10	3.44**

 * $p < .05$
** $p < .01$

REFERENCES

1. Danto BL: A bag full of laughs. *Amer J Psychiatry* 121:612-613, 1964.

2. Gonzalez EG, Downey JA: Polyneuropathy in a glue sniffer. *Arch Physical Med & Rehab* 53:333-337, 1972.

3. Goto I, et al: Toxic polyneuropathy due to glue sniffing. *J. Neurol Neurosurg & Psychiat* 37:848-853, 1974.

4. Grant WB: Inhalation of gasoline fumes by a child. *Psychiat Quarterly* 36:555, 1962.

5. Karani V: Peripheral neuritis after addiction to petrol. *British Med J* 1:216, 1966.

6. Mallov JS: MBK neuropathy among spray painters. *JAMA* 235:1455-1457, 1976.

7. Mitchell ABS, Parsons-Smith BG: Trichloroethylene neuropathy, *British Med J* 1:422-423, 1969.

8. Press E, Sterling J: Glue sniffing. Incidence, physiologic effects and police measures for controlling the inhalation of glue and other organic solvents. *Police* 12:14-20, 1968.

9. Chapel JL, Taylor DW: Glue sniffing. *Missouri Med* 65:288-292, 1968.

10. Faucett RL, Jensen RA: Addiction to the inhalation of gasoline fumes in a child. *J Pediatrics* 41:364-368, 1952.

11. Irwin W: *Drugs of Abuse*. Beloit, Student Association for the Study of Hallucinogens, 1970.

12. Louria DB: Medical complications of pleasure giving drugs. *Arch Int Med* 123:82, 1969.

13. Barman ML, et al: Acute and chronic effects of glue sniffing. *Cal Med* 100:19-22, 1964.

14. Brown NW: Gasoline inhalation. *J Med Assn Georgia* 57:217-221, 1968.

15. Dodds J, Santostefano S: A comparison of the cognitive functioning of glue-sniffers and non-sniffers. *J Pediatrics* 64:565-570, 1964.

16. James FM: The effects of cyclopropane anesthesia without surgical operation on mental functions of normal man. *Anesthesiology* 30:264-272, 1969.

17. Nylander I: Thinner-alcohol--Och tablettmissbruk bland barn och ungdom. *Nordic Medicine* 70:896-899, 1963.

18. Panse FR, Bender W: Toluol-xylol-psychose bei einem tiefdruckarbeiter. *Monatsschrift fuer Psychiatrie und Nuerologie* 89:249-259, 1934.

19. Halstead WC: *Brain and Intelligence: A Quantitative Study of the Frontal Lobes.* Chicago, University of Chicago Press, 1947.

20. Prockop LD: Huffer's neuropathy. *JAMA* 229:1083-1084, 1974.

21. Reitan RM: *The Effects of Brain Lesions on Adaptive Abilities in Human Beings.* Indianapolis, Privately published by the author, 1959.

22. Reitan RM: Verbal problem solving as related to cerebral damage. *Preceptual Motor Skills* 34:515-524, 1972.

23. Armitage SG: An analysis of certain psychological tests used for the evaluation of brain injury.

24. Berry GJ, et al: *Neuropsychological assessment of chronic inhalant abusers: A preliminary report. Proceedings of the First International Symposium on Voluntary Inhalation of Industrial Solvents.* In press, 1976.

25. Hathaway SR, McKinley JC: *The MMPI Manual.* Revised, New York, The Psychological Corporation, 1967.

26. Reitan RM: A research program on the psychological effects of brain lesions in human beings, in Ellis NR (ed): *International Review of Research in Mental Retardation, Vol. I.* New York, Academic Press, 1966.

27. Reitan RM: *Manual for Administration of Neuro-psychological Test Batteries for Adults and Children.* Indianapolis, Privately published by the author, 1969.

28. Reitan RM, Davison LA (eds): *Clinical Neuro-psychology: Current Status & Application.* New York, John Wiley & Sons, 1974.

29. Russell EW, et al: *Assessment of Brain Damage: A Neuropsychological Key Approach.* New York, John Wiley & Sons, 1970.

30. Saetveit JG, et al: Revision of the Seashore measures of musical talents. *Series on Aims and Progress of Research, No. 65.* Iowa City, University of Iowa Press, 1940.

31. Wechsler D: *Manual for the Wechsler Adult Intelligence Scale.* New York, The Psychological Corporation, 1955.

32. Wheeler L, Reitan RM: The presence and laterality
    of brain damage predicted from responses to a
    short aphasia screening test. *Perceptual Motor
    Skills* 15:783-799, 1962.

33. Dixon WJ, Massey FJ: *Introduction to Statistical
    Analysis*. New York, McGraw-Hill, 1957.

34. Carson RC: Interpretive manual to the MMPI, in
    Butcher JN (ed.): MMPI: *Research Developments and
    Clinical Applications*. New York, McGraw-Hill, 1969.

35. Dahlstrom WG, et al: *An MMPI Handbook. Volume I:
    Clinical Interpretation*. Minneapolis, University
    of Minnesota Press, 1972.

36. Marks PA, et al: *The Actuarial Use of the MMPI
    with Adolescents and Adults*. Baltimore, Williams
    & Wilkins Company, 1974.

37. Monachesi ED, Hathaway SR: The personality of
    delinquents, in Butcher JN (ed): *MMPI: Research
    Developments and Clinical Applications*. New York,
    McGraw-Hill, 1969.

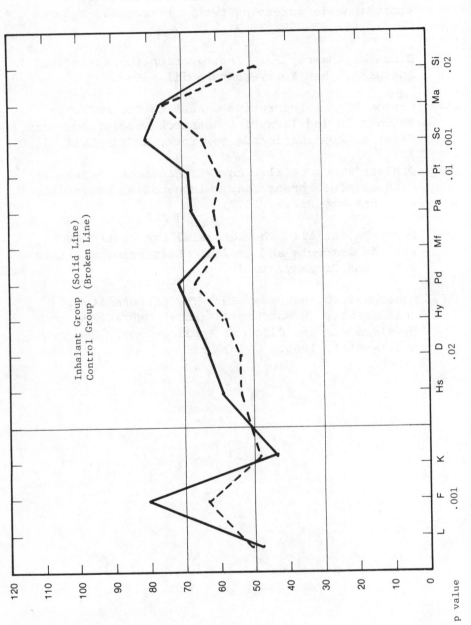

Figure 1. Minnesota Multiphasic Personality Inventory Mean Profiles for Inhalant and Control Groups

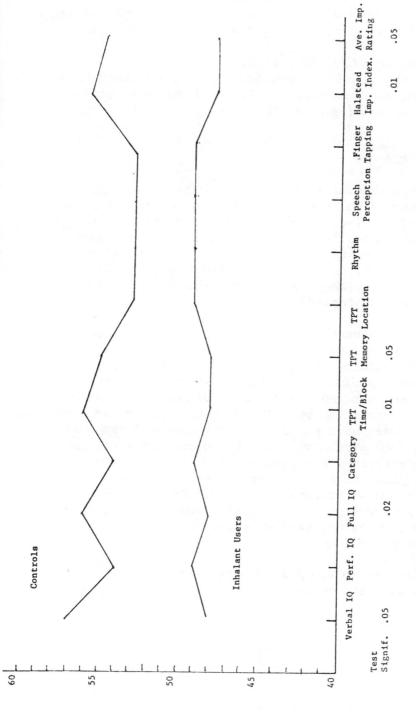

Figure 2. Standardized Scale Scores for WAIS I.Q. Values and Core Halstead Reitan Battery Tests*

*   Direction of scoring has been reversed for the Halstead Impairment Index, Category Test, Speech Sounds Perception and Time/Block.

HUMAN TOXICOLOGY OF POLYBROMINATED BIPHENYLS

Walter D. Meester, M.D., Ph.D.
*Director of Medical Research and Toxicology, Blodgett
Memorial Medical Center, Grand Rapids, Michigan*

Daniel J. McCoy, Sr., Ph.D.
*Associate Director, Clinical Toxicology Laboratory and
Analytical Toxicologist, Blodgett Memorial Medical
Center, Grand Rapids, Michigan*

ABSTRACT

*The erroneous mixing of approximately one ton of
polybrominated biphenyls (PBB), a commercial flame
retardant, into livestock feed in Michigan during mid-
1973 has resulted in one of the most costly agricultural accidents in the history of the United States.
As a result, hundreds of thousands of animals, including cattle, sheep, swine, and chickens have been destroyed and buried.*

*Although virtually every resident in Michigan has
been exposed to PBB-contaminated milk, meat, and eggs,
it is estimated that at least 2,000 farm families who
consumed products from their own PBB-contaminated farm
have received the heaviest exposure. Since March 1975
we have examined over 100 members of farm families who,
for an extended period of time, consumed PBB-contaminated food products. Over 60 subcutaneous fat biopsies
were performed to determine the concentration of PBB
in adipose tissue. Twenty biopsies were repeated after
a six-month interval. All patients were tested for
the presence of PBB in their blood. Control fat samples for PBB analysis were obtained from city and out-
of-state residents.*

*Although no specific disease entity or syndrome has
been ascribed to the effect of PBB, many of the indi-*

viduals we examined complained of easy fatigability,
muscle and joint pain, somnolence, easy irritability,
nervousness, headaches, visual problems, skin rashes,
decreased resistance to infections, decreased tolerance
to alcoholic beverages, and decreased libido. Some
patients presented with objective polymigratory arthri-
tis. One patient has aplastic anemia of undetermined
origin. Some patients are asymptomatic. A discussion
on the currently available clinical and laboratory data
on these patients will be presented.

The erroneous mixing of at least one ton of polybrominated biphenyls (PBB), a commercial flame retardant,
into livestock feed in Michigan during a period of at
least one year, starting sometime in mid-1973, has resulted in one of the most costly agricultural accidents
in the history of the United States. As a result, many
farms had to be quarantined and hundreds of thousands
of animals, including cattle, sheep, swine, and chickens,
have been destroyed and buried. The commercial name
of this chemical is Firemaster BP-6. It has an average
bromine content of six bromine atoms per biphenyl mol-
ecule. The mixture, however, also contains trace amounts
of tetra-, penta-, and heptabromobiphenyls. Recent GC
mass spectrometry analyses of the same fire retardant
by O'Keefe have shown that brominated benzenes, as well
as trace quantities of hexa-, and pentabromonaphthalene
also appear to be present. No dibenzofurans were detected in this product.

Cows which ingested the contaminated feed developed
anorexia and decreased milk production initially, followed by weight loss and the appearance of hematomas.
Abnormal growth of the hooves and alopecia also occurred.
Pregnant animals delivered two to four weeks late and
many calves were stillborn or died soon after birth.
Necropsy reports of cows which succumbed to the PBB
mixture mentioned liver changes, including fatty meta-
morphosis, large fat vacuoles replacing liver cells,

and amyloidosis. Acute, subacute, and chronic inter-
stitial mephritis was reported, and absomasal ulcers
were present in many animals. Numerous hematomas and
abscesses were also reported, as well as alopecia in
cattle, with abscess and ulcer formation on the udders,
swelling and redness of joints, and dead calves shortly
after birth. Many of the calves were born with extraordinarily large heads. The PBB contamination of the
livestock feed resulted in the consumption of this
chemical mixture by several million people through the
ingestion of contaminated meat and animal products.
The levels of consumption range from several thousand
parts per million in meat of contaminated dairy cows
to less than one part per million in milk sold in
supermarkets throughout the state. Virtually every
resident who has lived in the State of Michigan for
the last three years has been exposed to PBB-contaminated milk, meat, and eggs. It is estimated that at
least 2,000 farm families who consumed products from
their own PBB-contaminated farm have received the
heaviest exposure.

Although little is known about the toxicity of
polybrominated biphenyls, numerous deleterious effects
have been reported from a structurally similar group
of chemicals, the polychlorinated biphenyls. PCB's
are known to be embryo-lethal and cause reduction in
birth weights in rats. Teratogenicity has been demonstrated in chickens, and carcinogenic activity has been
reported in rats and mice. Enzyme induction as well as
injury to the cells has been demonstrated by PCB and
the immuno-suppressive activity of PCB is also well
documented. Furthermore, an outbreak of PCB poisoning,
known as the Yusho incident, occurred in Japan in 1968.
At least a thousand people were affected. Symptoms
included chloracne, blindness, gastrointestinal symptoms with jaundice, edema, and abdominal pain. Newborn
infants of the poisoned mothers had skin discoloration.
Also, decreased birth weight was noted.

Recent animal experiments with PBB have shown that
this agent is also a potent microsomal enzyme inducer
and has carcinogenic as well as teratogenic effects.
Other laboratory studies have shown that the potential
toxicity of the polybrominated biphenyls may be up to
five times that of the polychlorinated biphenyls.

In an attempt to evaluate the acute effects of PBB
exposure on human health, the Michigan Department of
Public Health began a study in the summer of 1974
involving 165 persons living on quarantined farms
(the exposed group) and 133 persons living on non-
quarantined farms (the control group). Medical histories were obtained by a written questionnaire and
about two-thirds of the subjects were examined by physical examination and routine urinalysis, complete blood
counts, and PBB blood levels. The persons selected for
the control group were presumably not exposed to PBB;
however, more than 70% of the subjects in the control
group had detectable levels of PBB in their blood. In
general, the blood values for PBB were higher in the
exposed group than in the control group. In this epidemiological study, symptoms were not considered to be
significant unless more than 10 individuals in the
study complained of them. Out of a group of 24 selected symptoms, illnesses, and complaints, only five
symptoms met this requirement. They were balance problems, rashes, headaches, fatigue, and anxiety. The
conclusion reached from this study was that there were
no acute or short term illnesses or pattern ailments
which could be clearly attributed to the exposure to
PBB. However, it was felt that the possible long-term-,
chronic-, or delayed effects of PBB on human health
remain to be answered. This study was valid in that
it compared individuals who lived on quarantined farms
to those who did not, but it was not a true comparison
between PBB exposed and unexposed individuals. Furthermore, the assumption that symptoms would not be significant unless more than 10 individuals complained about
them precluded discovery of potentially harmful problems

in a smaller number of individuals affected by PBB.
The assumption of the investigators that individuals
with the highest PBB blood levels should have more
symptoms than those with the lower blood levels, is
not necessarily true. It is well-known that blood
levels of highly fat soluble compounds are often inconsistent and unpredictable. Therefore, the assumption
that PBB levels in the blood are related to the severity
of signs and symptoms may be fallacious.

During the past year many farmers have been referred
to the Clinical Toxicology Service at Blodgett Hospital
for an evaluation of the possible toxic effects of PBB
on their health. As the year progressed, we have become more sophisticated in our evaluation. Whereas in
the beginning we only measured the presence of PBB in
the blood, it becomes rapidly apparent to us that a
more meaningful test, because of the compound's lipid
solubility, is the measurement of PBB in adipose tissue.
We found the mean level of PBB in a group of quarantined
farmers to be 1965 ppb as compared to a mean level of
516 ppb in non-quarantined farmers. City residents
had a mean level of 226 ppb whereas fat samples obtained
from a group of out-of-state residents were all negative
for PBB. There was a statistically significant difference at the 95% level of confidence between all of the
groups. So far, every person which we have tested who
has lived in the State of Michigan for the last three
years, has been found to have detectable levels of PBB
in their fat. To obtain comparative data on PBB levels
in paired specimens of fat and serum, a total of 116
subjects were tested. All subjects were positive for
PBB in their fat and the range of concentration of PBB
expressed in ppb was from a low of 58 to a high of
273,016 ppb. Only 35 of the paired serum samples were
positive for PBB, ranging in concentration from 0.1 ppb
to 28.6 ppb. The adipose tissue-serum ratios in these
35 individuals which were positive for PBB, both in
their fat and their serum, ranged from 27 to 14,850.
In other words, one individual had only 27 times the

amount of PBB in his fat as he had in his serum and
the individual at the high end had 14,850 times the
amount of PBB in his fat than he had in his serum.
The mean ratio, however, was 4,752. As compared to
earlier studies done by the Michigan Department of
Public Health, this ratio is significantly higher than
the ones obtained by them. This difference might be
due to the time difference in that many of the Michigan
Department of Public Health studies were done a year
earlier than ours and we have good evidence to show
that PBB blood levels are tapering off to very low or
near zero levels in PBB-exposed individuals. The lowest concentration of PBB in fat at which we found the
serum to be positive for PBB was 100 ppb and the highest concentration of PBB in fat at which we found serum
to be negative for PBB was 2391 ppb. There does not
appear to be a constant relationship between fat levels
of PBB and serum levels. In some individuals the fat
and serum levels seem to correlate but in others this
relationship is totally lacking. Undoubtedly, many
factors which affect lipolysis will affect the concentration of PBB in the blood, for example starvation,
exercise, cold exposure, smoking, diabetes, many drugs
and any adrenergic stimulation.

As time goes on, serum PBB levels appear to decrease.
Whereas during the last six months of 1975, we detected
many positive serum PBB levels averaging about two ppb,
during the first six months of this year we found many
individuals to be positive for PBB in their fat but
negative in their serum. The average PBB level in the
serum during the first six months of 1976 was ten times
lower than the average concentration during the last
six months of 1975. Figure 2 illustrates this a little
better in an individual in which one can see that the
fat levels of PBB which in October, 1974 was 13,000
ppb has decreased to 3690 ppb in February of 1976 and
his serum level of PBB has dropped from 23 ppb in
October of 1974 to only 1 ppb in February of 1976.
Just before I left for this meeting, I performed a

repeat fat biopsy on this individual and a venapuncture
for blood, and on the day I left, I was told that his
serum was negative now for PBB, whereas his fat level
has dropped to 1258 ppb. In contrast to the previous
patient, in this patient the fat level rose whereas the
serum level decreased (Figure 3). In addition to
serum and fat PBB levels, this person also had a
determination of PBB of his liver biopsy tissue as
well as of synovial fluid and bone marrow. As you can
see, his liver contained 300 ppb as compared to 1069
ppb in his fat and his synovial fluid only contained
twice the amount present in the serum whereas the
bone marrow contained only 3.5 ppb. We did a comparison of PBB levels in adipose tissue between husbands and wives. Biopsies of each were obtained on
the same day. Except for two of the 23 couples tested,
all of the husbands had a higher concentration of PBB
in their fat than their wives. The mean ratio was 2.4
with a standard error of 0.31. This means that males
on the average have 2½ times the levels of PBB in their
fat as females. We also discovered that children often
had higher levels than their parents. We feel that the
level of PBB in fat is related to the total amount of
fat present in a person and the relative amount of
adipose tissue in females is greater than in males
whereas the relative amount of adipose tissue present
in children is less than that of adults. It should be
apparent from these findings that the setting of a
tolerance level of .3 ppm in cattle may be an arbitrary
one. It also points out that adipose tissue PBB determinations without an assessment of a person's weight
and an estimate of the total amount of adipose tissue
present may not reflect a true measurement of the total
amount of PBB present in the body.

PBB is excreted in human milk. This study was done
by Humphrey and Hayner during the latter part of 1974
and the early part of 1975 at which time blood PBB
levels in some individuals undoubtedly were still very
high. In a more recent assessment of the excretion of

PBB in human milk as well as the transfer of PBB to the fetus, we found that in mothers who have low levels of PBB in their fat and who are negative for PBB in their serum, there is no PBB detected in their breast milk nor in the cord blood, amniotic fluid, or placental or cord tissue. We have not yet examined any mothers who have very high levels of PBB in their fat. Currently, we have two of these in our study group but they have not yet delivered a baby. The findings depicted show that women in the State of Michigan who have low levels of PBB do not have to unnecessarily worry about PBB present in their milk, and it is our recommendation that mothers with low levels of PBB in their fat should be encouraged, if they would like to do so, to nurse their babies.

In an attempt to evaluate the time of exposure to PBB contaminated food products and its relationship to concentrations of PBB in fat, we obtained serum and fat specimens from volunteer foreign students who have resided in the State of Michigan for one year, two years, and three years. None of the students were positive for PBB in their serum and the students who had lived in Michigan for the past year were also negative for PBB in their fat. Those who had resided in the State of Michigan for two years had low levels of PBB in their fat and the group of students who resided in Michigan for the past three years had considerably higher levels of PBB in their fat. From these observations it might be concluded that the heaviest exposure to PBB to the residents in the State of Michigan was during the year that the PBB contamination of livestock feed went undetected. I should add here that the erroneous mixing of PBB with livestock allegedly first occurred in May of 1973 and was not detected until a year later.

We performed repeat fat biopsies on a number of individuals and found that the average decrease in concentration of PBB in a period of six months was about 40%. All of these repeat biopsies were performed within the last couple of months and in every one of the subjects tested there was a significant decrease in the PBB level.

Figure 4 shows the decrease in PBB levels in serum of three members of the same family. Whereas back in October of 1974 there still appeared to be an increase in serum levels in two members of this family, by February of 1976 the serum levels have diminished significantly, in spite of the fact that this family has extremely high PBB levels in their fat. As a matter of fact, this 14-year-old boy has the highest level which we have measured, namely 273,000 ppb. He seems in apparent good health and has not developed any specific disease. Figure 5 shows serum PBB levels in three members of another family and again, it shows marked decreases in serum PBB levels whereas the fat levels in these individuals are still very high.

I think it should be clear from the data I have presented so far that many people in the State of Michigan have ingested food contaminated with PBB. The farmers who had a problem with PBB on their farms have obviously received the heaviest exposure. The period of heavy exposure was undoubtedly during the year that the contamination went undetected, that is from May of 1973 to May of 1974. The rate of excretion of the chemical is undoubtedly faster than was originally anticipated, although, compared to other chemicals it does seem to have a relatively long half life. Clinical studies to determine the effects of PBB on man can obviously not be performed in a prospective way and are by necessity retrospective in nature. For this reason it may not be possible for anyone to definitively show the existence of a specific syndrome unless another similar disaster should occur. The Michigan Department of Public Health clinical studies were carried out more than a year after the first contamination occurred and our evaluation of patients more than two years

after the accident occurred. Naturally these studies
are useful to uncover any delayed and long term effects. However, the acute effects may not be apparent
anymore.

Nevertheless, we made an attempt to uncover any specific disease entity or syndrome which might have been
associated with the acute exposure of PBB and we found
a number of symptoms which were most prevalent in the
patients we have seen. We compared the percent of
occurrence of symptoms in the group of quarantined
farmers with non-quarantined farmers and also with
those who had fat PBB levels greater than 2,000 ppb.
These groups were also compared with the group at
large, i.e. the total group. We observed that more
than half of the patients complained of extreme tired-
ness and easy fatigability. This was consistent in
all of the groups. The next most common symptom was
that of joint pain. About 40% of the patients complained about pain in their joints usually in their
extremities. Many of these arthralgias were polymigratory in nature. The next most common symptom
was that of headache; then muscle pain, dizziness,
backache, joint stiffness, blurred vision somnolence,
nervousness, rash and these rashes varied in kind,
however, four people in the group had acne like rashes.
Seventeen percent complained about abdominal pain, 11
and 10% respectively of irritability and diarrhea.
There is no statistical significant difference between
the incidence of symptoms in any one of these four
groups.

Other symptoms less frequently encountered included
alcohol intolerance, decreased resistance, decreased
libido, depression, muscle weakness, numbness and
tingling, pruritis, sores of the mucous membranes,
weight loss and coordination problems. In many instances the onset of symptoms in individual patients
dated back to the fall of 1973 or the early part of
1974. Many patients have told me they are gradually

feeling better. Also several patients are completely
asymptomatic and have been asymptomatic during the
past three years. In the way of clinical findings,
we observed 14 patients to have exogenous obesity,
8 patients with dermatitis, 3 of which had an acne-
form like rash; 7 patients were hypertensive; 6 patients had objective type of arthritis, 2 of which
could be contributed to gout, one to rheumatoid arthritis and 3 of them had rheumatoid-like arthritis
with negative rheumatoid factor. Five of them had
evidence of bony exostosis. Four patients presented
with subcutaneous lipomatous lesions. Three of the
men had prostatic hypertrophy. Three of the women
were pregnant. Three cardiac murmers were heard.
Two patients had inguinal hernias. Two patients had
nail anomalies with pitting of the nails. Two patients had varicose veins. Two patients presented
with pretibial edema. Two patients suffered from
severe depression and one patient was schizophrenic
with symptoms of paranoia. One patient had a peripheral neuropathy for which other causes such as
diabetes and heavy metal poisoning were ruled out.
This neuropathy appears to be a reversible one in
that the patient during the past year has experienced
marked improvement. One patient presented with
Raynaud's disease; another patient referred to us had
aplastic anemia which developed about two years ago.
One patient was hypothyroid; another patient had
exophthalmos thought to be due to endocrine causes.
One patient had mastitis; another had a scrotal
lesion which turned out to be a benign epididymal
cyst. One patient presented with mastoiditis, another patient had a pilonidal cyst and one of the
patients was recently diagnosed to have a gastric
adenocarcinoma.

In as far as laboratory tests are concerned we did
not perform a standard set of tests on each patient.
We only performed those tests which at the time of
physical examination were felt to be indicated. The

reason for this is that although we attempted a clinical evaluation of the possible toxicity of PBB, we did
not have any research monies to absorb the cost of ex-
pensive laboratory evaluations. In a number of patients
we performed liver enzyme profiles including serum gam-
ma glutamic transpeptidase, alkaline phosphatase-, and
LDH isoenzymes. In a small number of patients we also
performed coagulation studies and serum immunoglobulins.
In only four patients did we find abnormal elevations
of liver isoenzymes. In one of the patients who exhibited objective polymigratory arthritis we found
borderline abnormal liver enzymes changes, and his
liver biopsy showed minimal focal necrosis and liver
cell drop-out. This patient's liver parenchyma reveals occasional random focus of drop-out of liver
cells, associated with minimal focal reactive changes.
A higher magnification shows an occasional binucleate
liver cell and an occasional clear nucleus suggestive
of accumulation of glycogen. Bone marrow examination
of this same patient showed significant increase in
absolute reticulocyte count and occasional erythroblast
islands in the bone marrow tissue suggesting a possible
autoimmune hemolytic component. Subsequently, a class-
specific hyperglobulinemia was ruled out in this patient.

Among the findings was an acne-like rash on the
chest of a patient who reported he had this type of
rash on different parts of his body for the past two
years. There was also an acne-like rash on a gentle-
man who reported having severe difficulty raising his
arm for the past two years. A farmer reported that
he had been wading in the feed when feeding his livestock. He claims he wore high boots but since June
of 1973 he has had a rash on his legs. On examination
his skin condition showed hyperkeratosis and discoloration. This man also has varicose veins.

It is impossible at this stage of the game to say
with any degree of certainty that PBB was responsible

for any of the findings which I have presented to you today. Obviously, in a retrospective evaluation such as this, a clear cut cause and effect relationship can never be proven. Many of the symptoms and complaints could be of psychosomatic origin and undoubtly many of the farmers affected by PBB contamination of their livestock have suffered great losses and thus may be affected psychologically. In the personal evaluation of the patients we always carefully tried to differentiate between psychogenic symptoms and other symptoms which might be caused by organic disease. In my mind the most outstanding symptoms involve the skeletoneuromuscular system. The fact that several people who presented with joint and muscle pain which they never experienced before and were found to have objective type of arthritis suggests that with all other causes ruled out, that PBB might be responsible or may have contributed to their problems. Also, the patient with an unexplained peripheral neuropathy, the onset of which coincided with the exposure to PBB, suggests a possible relationship. Babies born so far to mothers exposed to PBB appear to have been normal except for one baby we know of who was born with club feet. However, the overall rate of fetal abnormalities in the general population is 2% and it will be impossible to prove a relationship between PBB and fetal anomalies in so small a series of cases.

I would like to close with some recommendations with regards to the future evaluation of the effect of polybrominatedbiphenyls:

1. Continued clinical evaluation and long-term follow-up of patients known to have ingested large amounts of PBB as documented by history and fat biopsies. These patients to undergo periodic complete clinical and laboratory evaluation and long-term follow-up. The examinations to include an evaluation of hepatic and renal function, collagen and immune response studies, fertility studies, PBB excretion

studies, neuromuscular system studies, evaluation of
the development of malignant neoplasms or other tumor-
like lesions, evaluation of the offspring born to
women with high levels of PBB, evaluation of alcohol
and drug interactions, side effects, and other studies
deemed necessary to completely evaluate the possible
effects of PBB on any organ system which might be
affected.

2. Laboratory studies on the carcinogenicity,
mutagenicity, and teratogenicity of PBB in animals
as well as in human tissue cultures.

3. Laboratory studies on the absorption, metabolism/
degradation, and excretion of PBB in primates and other
laboratory animals.

4. An epidemiological study on the incidence of
spontaneous abortions, infertility, rate of fetal
anomalies, incidence of cancer, and other possible
parameters occuring in the population at large in the
State of Michigan as compared to the population of
another industrial state free of PBB. This is to be
a long-term study, continuing for at least 20 years.

5. Studies to develop methods, mechanisms, or
drugs to facilitate degradations and/or excretion of
PBB to lower body levels.

6. An evaluation of possible toxic effects of PBB
contaminants such as naphthalene.

7. Studies on the interactions between PBB and
other chemical substances, such as alcohol and drugs,
especially those which are known to induce hepatic
microsomal enzymes.

TABLE I

PBB LEVELS IN ADIPOSE TISSUE

GROUP	CONCENTRATION IN P.P.B. (MEAN ± S.E.)
Quarantined Farmers	1965* ± 356 (N = 53)
Non-quarantined Farmers	516* ± 92 (N = 29)
City Residents	226* ± 73 (N = 9)
Out-of-state Residents	Neg. (N = 20)

*Indicates a statistically significant difference (P < 0.05) from the other groups.

TABLE II

COMPARATIVE DATA ON PBB LEVELS IN PAIRED
SPECIMENS OF HUMAN ADIPOSE TISSUE AND SERUM
(April 1, 1975 - June 30, 1976)

Number of subjects   116

PBB positive fat samples   116
    Range of concentration (ppb)   58 - 273,016

PBB positive serum samples   35
    Range of concentration (ppb)   0.1 - 28.6

Adipose tissue - serum ratios (N = 35)
    Range   27 - 14,850
    Mean ± SE   4,752 ± 793

Lowest concentration (ppb) in fat at
    which serum positive for PBB   100

Highest concentration (ppb) in fat at
    which serum negative for PBB   2,391

TABLE III

COMPARISON OF SERUM PBB LEVELS

Time Period	Concentration in ppb (Mean ± SE)
June 1, 1975-- Dec. 31, 1975	2.0 ± 0.33 (N = 56)
Jan. 1, 1976-- June 30, 1976	0.2 ± 0.05 (N = 77)

TABLE IV

COMPARISON OF PBB LEVELS IN ADIPOSE TISSUE

Date of Subc. Fat Biopsies	Concentration in P.P.B.		Ratio H/W
	Husband	Wife	
12-10-75	9468	4043	2.34
1-14-76	710	396	1.79
1-28-76	673	305	2.21
1-28-76	410	352	1.16
2-02-76	1561	987	1.58
2-05-76	4967	3844	1.29
2-12-76	2280	463	4.92
2-12-76	246	113	2.18
2-12-76	826	345	2.39
2-26-76	1167	236	4.94
3-11-76	1374	869	1.58
3-24-76	188	58	3.24
3-25-76	7605	1525	4.99
3-25-76	6116	5139	1.19
3-31-76	343	239	1.44
3-31-76	129	255	0.51
4-01-76	321	310	1.04
4-01-76	659	380	1.73
4-03-76	146040	26519	5.51
4-21-76	1454	650	2.24
4-21-76	1624	400	4.06
4-28-76	193	277	0.70
5-17-76	1044	508	2.06

$$\overline{X} = 2.40$$

$$SE = 0.31$$

TABLE V

COMPARISON OF PBB CONCENTRATIONS IN
HUMAN BREAST MILK AND BLOOD PLASMA*

Subject	Date	PBB Levels (ppm) Breast Milk	Blood Plasma
E.B.	12/74	10.800	.082
C.M.	06/74	22.700	.252
D.S.	10/74	1.800	.014
L.H.	03/75	.210	.003
S.S.	03/75	92.660	1.068

*Humphrey and Hayner, Proceedings of the 9th Annual
Conference on Trace Substances in Environmental
Health, June 1975.

TABLE VI

PBB LEVELS AFTER GESTATION (in ppb)

Mother's		Breast	Cord	Amniotic	Placental or
Serum	Fat	Milk	Blood	Fluid	Cord Tissue
0	185	0	0	–	0
0	234	0	0	0	0
0	345	0	0	0	0

TABLE VII

PBB LEVELS IN FOREIGN STUDENTS*

Living in Michigan for the Past:	Concentration in ppb (Mean $\pm$ SE)	
	In Fat:	In Serum
1 Year (N = 5)	Neg	Neg
2 Years (N = 5)	82 $\pm$ 34	Neg
3 Years (N = 5)	1000 $\pm$ 209	Neg

*Tests done in May 1976.

TABLE VIII

PBB LEVELS IN MAN AFTER SIX-MONTH INTERVAL

| Subject's | | Concentration in ppb | | Percent |
Age	Sex	First Fat Biopsy	Repeat Biopsy	Change
37	M	359	100	↓ 72%
39	M	666	593	↓ 11%
44	M	9468	2617	↓ 72%
42	F	4043	2919	↓ 28%
20	M	12716	5411	↓ 57%
9	F	5425	3003	↓ 45%
25	F	2115	1023	↓ 52%
28	M	1461	1044	↓ 29%
51	M	485	239	↓ 51%
24	F	881	752	↓ 15%
32	M	1226	879	↓ 28%
9	M	710	612	↓ 14%
32	F	396	175	↓ 56%
11	F	508	336	↓ 34%
42	M	410	254	↓ 38%
66	M	673	507	↓ 25%

$$\chi = \downarrow 39\%$$

TABLE IX

PERCENT OCCURRENCE OF SYMPTOMS IN VARIOUS GROUPS OF MEMBERS
OF MICHIGAN FARM FAMILIES EXPOSED TO PBB.

Symptom	Total Group 1452±223* (N=82)	Quarantined Farmers 1965±356* (N=53)	Non-Quarantined Farmers 516±92* (N=29)	Farmers With PBB Levels <2000 (N=21)
Fatigue	55	51	65	61
Joint Pain	38	41	34	38
Headache	31	34	24	38
Muscle Pain	24	24	24	24
Dizziness	20	19	24	24
Backache	19	20	17	24
Joint Stiffness	19	19	20	19
Blurred Vision	17	15	20	19
Somnolence	17	17	17	24
Nervousness	16	20	10	14
Skin Rash	15	15	14	24
Abdominal Pain	17	14	24	14
Irritability	11	10	14	10
Diarrhea	10	10	10	9

*Mean Concentration (±S.E.) of PBB in Subcutaneous Adipose Tissue.

TABLE X

OTHER SYMPTOMS LESS FREQUENTLY ENCOUNTERED

Alcohol Intolerance

Decreased Resistance

Decreased Libido

Depression

Muscle Weakness

Numbness and Tingling

Pruritis

Sores of Mucous Membranes

Weight Loss

Balance Problems

TABLE XI

CLINICAL FINDINGS IN MEMBERS OF FARM
FAMILIES EXPOSED TO PBB.
(49 Males; 33 Females; 14 Children)

Obesity	14	Depression	2
Dermatitis	8	Schizophrenia	1
Hypertension	7	Periph. Neuropathy	1
Arthritis	6	Raynaud's Disease	1
Exostosis	5	Aplastic Anemia	1
Lipomatosis	4	Hypothyroidism	1
Prostatic Hypertrophy	3	Exophthalmos	1
Pregnancy	3	Mastitis	1
Cardiac Murmur	3	Epididymal Cyst	1
Inguinal Hernia	2	Mastoiditis	1
Pitted Nails	2	Pilonidal Cyst	1
Varicose Veins	2	Gastric Adenocarcinoma	1
Pretibial Edema	2		

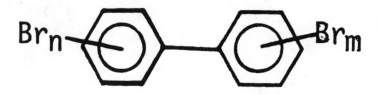

Figure 1. Polybrominated Biphenyls (PBB)

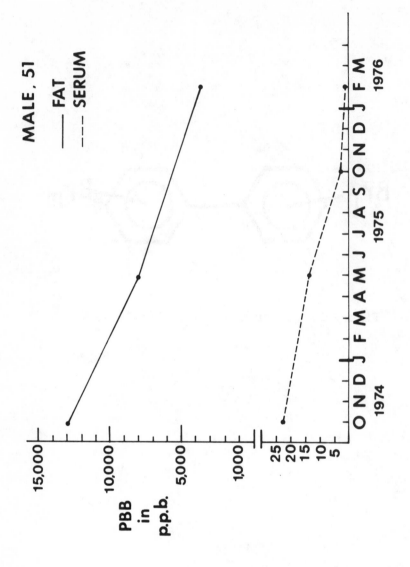

Figure 2. PPB Level v. Time

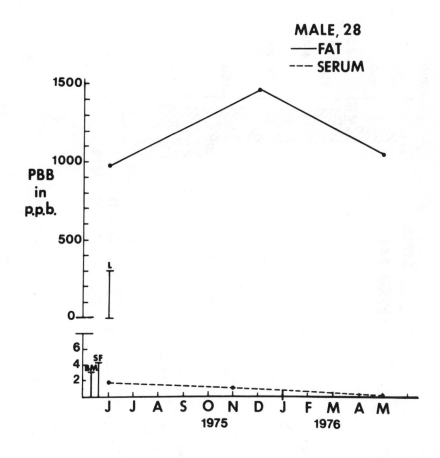

Figure 3. PPB Level v. Time

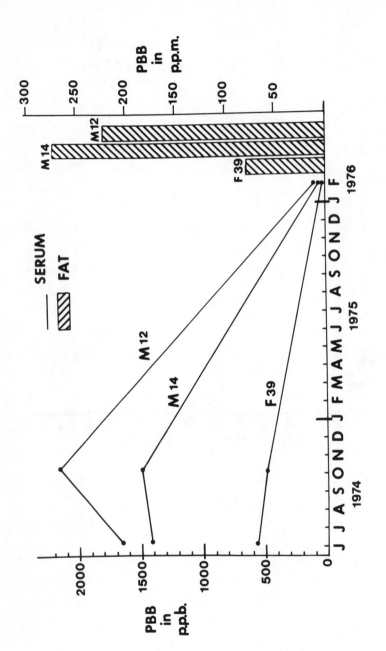

Figure 4. PPB Level v. Time

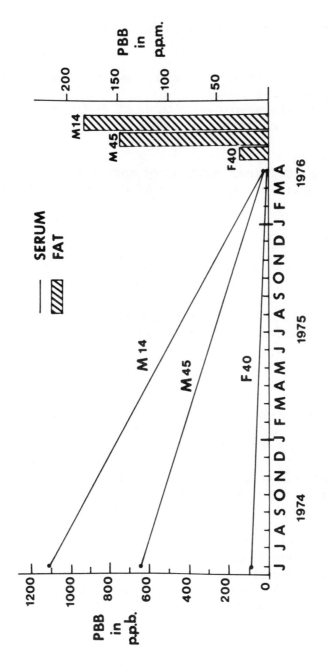

Figure 5. PBB Level v. Time

THE TRICYCLIC ANTIDEPRESSANT OVERDOSED PATIENT

W.D. Winters, M.D., Ph.D.
Director, Poison Control Center, Emergency Medicine,
Sacramento Medical Center
Professor of Pharmacology, School of Medicine,
University of California at Davis

M. Johnson, M.D.
Professor of Clinical Psychiatry and Pharmacology,
School of Medicine, University of California at Davis

ABSTRACT

A review of 25 patients that overdosed on tricyclic antidepressants (TCA) indicated that the typical patient was a 28-year-old female that ingested 1.5 gm of amitriptyline, along with a hypnotic or alcohol. 50% of the patients had an arrhythmia and/or heart block; 11 had a HR of 140 or greater, 12 had an admission systolic greater than 140, and 9 had a systolic less than 100.

The patients entered with one of three types of symptoms: 1) history of ingestion but no symptoms except a mild tachycardia; 2) coma and/or convulsion with elevated BP and HR greater than 140; 3) coma and occasionally convulsions with reduced BP and HR of 120 or less. Nine patients with type 2 went on to type 3, six patients with type 1 went on to type 2 or 3. The duration of type 1 is about 2 hours, type 2 is about 1-4 hours, and type 3 usually occurs within 4 hours of ingestion if untreated. Since the TCA are muscarinic blocking agents, it appears that the latency of type 1 can be related to delayed gastric emptying into the duodenum where maximal TCA absorption occurs. Type 2 appears to be related to the NE reuptake blocking properties of TCA inducing excessive $\propto$ and β adrenergic stimulation resulting in increased HR and BP. The type

3 effect appears to occur when the catecholes wash out of synaptic areas and there is a depletion of α sympathetic tone. The effective reversal of the arrhythmias, heart block, and increase of the decreased BP, by physostigmine suggests that the TCA exerts a cholinergic block on the NE reuptake system as well as a vagolytic action.

How much of each type of TCA reaction is observed after admission appears to be related to the dose ingested, time to removal of G.I. contents, treatment regimen, and other drugs ingested. The use of physostigmine and the correction of acidosis with bicarbonate are essential for successful treatment of severe TCA overdoses (three cases required pacemakers). There does not appear to be any significant difference in severity of symptoms or duration of action between the various TCA agents ingested, including doxepin.

INTRODUCTION

There has been a marked increase in the use of tricyclic antidepressant drugs during the past ten years. The treatment indications include psychotic depression, enuresis, underachieving and behavior problems, and in the treatment of drug dependence induced depression. The antidepressant drugs include imipramine (Tofranil), amitriptyline (Elavil), desipramine (Norpramine), nortriptyline (Aventyl), and doxepine (Sinequan). These agents are often used in combination with benzdiazepines, phenothiazines, sedatives, hypnotics, or alcohol. The tricyclics are basic drugs which are structurally similar to the phenothiazines. Therapeutic actions are not evident in less than five to seven days and there is a residual action after the drug use has ceased. The prolonged action is partially based on the large volume of distribution ($VD > 30$ L/Kg) with a slow washout from the body ($t_{1/2}$ 30-50 hrs).

The major pharmacological actions are related to
their antidepressant, anticholinergic and antihista-
minic actions, as well as the block of the reuptake
of released norepinephrine. In addition, they have
a quinidine-like effect on the heart which may be of
an anticholinergic action. The anticholinergic action
of these compounds may cause symptoms such as dryness
of mouth, blurred vision, constipation, and urinary
retention. Disorientation and mental confusion may
also be related to the central anticholinergic effect
of these agents. Sedation may be considerable even
in therapeutic doses and these drugs are often used
in a single dose at bedtime for this reason. The
antihistamic actions of these drugs are of no practical
clinical importance. Cardiovascular side effects
include tachycardia, arrhythmias, and prolongation of
the atrioventricular conduction time. The interference
with nerepinephrine uptake may explain many of these
effects.

OVERDOSAGE

The first report of imipramine overdose death
appeared in 1961 and the first report of amitriptyline
overdose death occurred in 1965. Since that time there
has been an increasing number of patients overdosing on
these agents. Overdose from these agents can be divided
into two main categories, namely; 1) accidental, which
occurs usually in children, and 2) suicide attempts by
adult patients incompletely treated for depression.
Toxicity is usually noted in adults who ingest over
500 mg per day; the average dose for ingestion at our
hospital is 1.3 gm and some patients have consumed over
2.5 gm and survived with early treatment.

Based on the clinical symptoms it is possible to
describe a continuum of effects following excessive
doses of tricyclic antidepressants and to divide these
into four specific stages.

Stage 1. - Latent stage.

Since these agents are basic compounds they are present in the ionized form in the stomach and therefore not absorbed until they enter the alkaline midportion of the duodeum. In addition, these agents have anticholinergic action which blocks cholinergic receptors within the stomach and intestine (Fig. 1). As a result of this local action on the musculature of the upper G.I. tract there is a delay in gastric motility and emptying. Thus the ionized drug remains in the stomach for prolonged periods of time and there is some time following the ingestion before systemic symptoms become manifest. The time since last eating, the number of pills taken, and the volume of fluid taken with the pills are a few of the variables which determine the duration of this latent period. In general this latent period lasts between 1/2 - 1-1/2 hours postingestion. Towards the end of this stage as some drug is absorbed into the peripheral circulation, systemic effects of the anticholinergic properties of this drug will become manifest; such as, dryness of mouth, slight dilatation of the pupils, and sinus tachycardia up to approximately 120 beats per minute (vagal block). As this stage progresses, excitation, hallucinations, disorientation, or confusion may become manifest.

Stage 2. - Catechol inhanced effect.

During Stage 2 the effects of the block of the reuptake of norepinephrine in sympathetic nerve endings become apparent. These effects are manifest by enhanced α and β receptor stimulation (see Fig. 2). The α effects will be on the pressor receptors of blood vessels and the β_1 effects will be noted on cardiac rate and excitability. Symptoms during this stage include tachycardia beyond 120 beats per minute, increased blood pressure - both systolic and diasystolic, cardiac arrhythmias, first degree AV block, right or

left bundlebranch block; increasing in severity to
complete AV block, ventricular tachycardia, ventricular
fibrillation and cardiac arrest. In addition during
this phase patients may manifest increased temperature,
coma (see Table 1 for coma stages), and/or convulsions.
This stage lasts approximately two hours and if untreated
will progress to Stage 3.

Stage 3. - Partial catechol depletion.

During this stage released catecholamines which are
no longer capable of being taken back into the neuron
are degraded by the slow turnover enzyme catechol-o-
methyl transferase (COM-T) and/or diffuse out of the
synaptic spaces. There will be a reduction in the
number of occupied receptors at sympathetic nerve
endings. As a result the blood pressure falls to
shock level and the heart rate drops to approximately
100. If the blood pressure is below 60/40 and the
depletion of catechols in the heart are significant,
the heart rate may fall to below 40. During this
stage the arrhythmias and block that began during
Stage 2 continue or become more serious; i.e. complete
heart block, PVC, ventricular tachycardia, fibrillation
or arrest. The stage of coma (2-3) becomes increasingly
deeper and convulsions may continue to occur. If this
stage is not adequately treated the patient will continue to a more profound depth of coma (4) and cardiovascular status characterized by the next stage.

Stage 4. - Complete catechol washout.

As the washout of catecholamines progresses to the
point where essentially all NE is depleted from synaptic spaces, the level of sympathetic tone in the α
receptors disappears and the patient will manifest a
complete loss of blood pressure. In addition, the
complete loss of NE for β_1 stimulation of the heart
will result in the heart rate dropping to complete
arrest or the occurrence of ventricular arrhythmias.

At this time there is complete pump failure and electrical stimulation may not be effective in reversing the ventrical arrhythmias or a pacer may not be effective for heart block. If this condition is not properly, rapidly, and adequately treated this stage will be irreversible.

TREATMENT

The most important initial principle in the treatment of the tricyclic antidepressant overdose is to prevent the absorption of that portion of the drug which still remains in the gastrointestinal tract. The techniques involve emesis or lavage, activated charcoal adsorption, and catharsis. The decision between emesis and lavage depends on the accuracy of the initial history and the duration between the time the patient is seen and the time that the drug was initially ingested. Usually if a significant amount of drug was ingested and it occurred one hour or more prior to admission, even in the presence of an intact gag reflex, the patient should be intubated and lavaged. If however the patient is seen early, that is within 45 minutes of the time of ingestion, and has an intact gag reflex, a trial dose of 30 ml of Ipecac Syrup can be attempted. If within 20-30 minutes after Ipecac the patient does not have an emesis the patient should be lavaged. Under no circumstances should these patients receive a second dose of Ipecac. If the decision is made to intubate the patient in the presence of a gag reflex, it is often necessary to seek the aid of an anesthesist to paralyze the vocal cords to prevent the induction of laryngeal spasm or trauma. In the presence of a gag reflex it is possible to pass a large bore lavage tube into the stomach with a minimum hazard to the respiratory tree. However, one cannot be certain that during the total period of lavage the gag reflex will remain intact and therefore this procedure is more hazardous. Placing the patient in the head down left recumbent position makes this procedure somewhat safer

however, it does not completely protect the airway.
Following emptying of the stomach contents, 30-50
grams of activated charcoal in a slurry should be administered orally followed by a cathartic. Either
magnesium or sodium sulfate are adequate cathartics
for catharsis.

Since the tricyclic antidepressants are basic compounds having a large volume distribution the distribution is markedly in favor of entry into cells at the
expense of plasma concentration. Plasma levels are low
and may be below the level of sensitivity of the laboratory analysis, therefore urine chromatography may be
the best method of detection. In cells the compounds
are ion trapped and thus do not readily diffuse back
to the plasma. As a result there is little benefit
in attempting to reduce body content of these agents
by either peritoneal or hemodialysis. Acidification
of the urine might enhance the clearance of this drug
through the kidney, however there are no studies to
substantiate this procedure. In addition, acidification runs the risk of increasing the sensitivity of
the myocardium to arrhythmias. In fact there is literature indicating that the myocardium is most protected in a state of plasma alkalosis. There are no
demonstrated techniques for increasing the rate of
metabolism of the drug in the body thus once the drug
enters the body it is slowly removed.

There are several reports indicating that the duration of action of the tricyclic antidepressant drug
can be reduced by utilization of continuous or periodic
gastric suction. The administration of pulses of
activated charcoal have been effective in reducing
the duration of the tricyclic action in experimental
animals. The rational for this technique is related
to the fact that the tricyclics are basic drugs and
are ion trapped in the acid secretions entering the
stomach. Gastric suction and/or adsorbtion to activated charcoal would remove the drug present in the

stomach. If not removed from the stomach they will
pass into the duodeum, become unionized in the alkaline portion and be reabsorbed.

Since the tricyclic antidepressant agents manifest
profound anticholinergic action, especially in overdose situations, it is possible to reverse many of
these symptoms by administeration of a cholinesterase
inhibitor. The dose of the cholinesterase inhibitor
must be titrated against the degree of muscarinic
blocking by the tricyclic antidepressant, therefore
it is preferable to use a short acting cholinesterase
reversible inhibitor rather than an irreversible inhibitor such as the organophosphates. The carbamate
colinesterase inhibitors are short acting and reversible and are therefore most useful in the tricyclic
toxic state. Since symptoms of toxicity involve
both CNS and cardiovascular systems it is necessary
to administer a carbamate which is capable of
crossing both the blood brain barrier and tissue
membrane in the peripheral tissues. Most carbamate cholinesterase inhibitors like prostigmine and
edrophonium are quarternary ammonium salts so that
at blood pH they are in the ionized form and will not
easily or effectively cross the blood brain barrier.
Physostigmine is a tertiary ammonium compound, is
unionized at neutral pH in serum and thus will effectively cross the blood brain barrier and is the drug
of choice in dealing with these situations.

Indications for the use of physostigmine are deep
coma, convulsions, hyperpyrexia, tachycardia above
140, hypertension, hypotension, cardiac arrhythmias,
AV and bundlebranch block and pump failure. The
usual dosage in the adult is 1-2 mg given intravenously
slowly over a period of at least one minute. The
latency to effect is approximately 10-15 minutes. It
is important to do a complete assessment of the patient
prior to administration of physostigmine and then follow
the course of the patient after the physostigmine, for

about 1/2 hour to evaluate the effectiveness of the physostigmine. The latency to the onset of effect is based on the fact that inhibition of cholinesterase, per se, will not reverse the effect of the anticholinergic action of the tricyclic antidepressant; it is necessary for the acetylcholine levels in synaptic areas to build up to effective levels to reverse the muscarinic block.

Some patients will enter the Emergency Department with seizures and some may develop seizures following administration of physostigmine. The literature is not clear in terms of evaluating the role of physostigmine in inducing or blocking the seizures. If there is evidence that there is a correlation between the time course of the administration of physostigmine and the development of convulsions, physostigmine should be used cautiously. It may be necessary to use a quarternary ammonium cholinesterase inhibitor to deal with the peripheral cardiovascular problems rather than continue to use the physostigmine if it is strongly implicated as the cause of the seizures in a patient. Seizures if not controlled by physostigmine should be treated by the use of either intravenous doses of diazepam or a short acting barbiturate.

The cardiovascular problems resulting from tricyclic overdosage will respond to physostigmine in most cases. Lidocaine (xylocaine) should be used cautiously since it may potentiate the anticholinergic and quinidine-like actions of tricyclics during toxicity. Alkalinization of the blood using intravenous sodium bicarbonate has been reported by both the French and Australians to be effective in reducing the excitability of the myocardium in this toxic state. Additionally phentoin has been reported to be effective in reducing arrhythmias and as a last resort could be tried. Propranolol should only be used in serious sinus tachycardia which does not respond to physostigmine. The problem with propranolol is that if the patient progresses to Stage 4. - Catechol washout, it would be very difficult to activate the β receptors of the myocardium in the presence of the β block. A demand pacemaker should be available and utilized if necessary if the patient does not respond to physostigmine in the presence of heart block. Defibrillation is indicated in the presence of ventricular tachycardia or fibrillation. If the heart does not respond to electrical stimulation as in pump failure this indicates that there is a complete loss of catechol from the myocardium. Prior to continuing electrical stimulation it is necessary to administer a β agonist agent like norepinephrine or isoproterenol to support the excitability of the heart. If there is peripheral vascular collapse then an α agonist such as norepinephrine or dopamine would be necessary to raise the blood pressure. Norepinephrine may have enough β action along with its α stimulating action to perform both the replenishment of the α and β depleted catechol stores and should be tried prior to the using of isoproterenol in the presence of both pump failure and peripheral vascular collapse. It is important to use physostigmine in the presence of pump failure as well as alkalinization since physostigmine appears to reverse the tricyclic block of the reuptake of catecholamines back into synapses. By replenishing the catecholamines and enhancing reuptake back into presynaptic endings the normalization of the physiological status of the synapse seems to occur and may significantly reduce the dose of norepinephrine administered for α and β function.

The role of physostigmine in the reversal of the tricyclic block of catecholamine reuptake is possibly based on a cholinergic role in the reuptake system. Further studies are necessary to clarify this theory.

In terms of the protocol for monitoring patients it is recommended that all tricyclic or anticholinergic containing ingestions be monitored in the hospital if it is ascertained that a significant ingestion has

occurred. Patients who have CNS or anticholinergic
symptoms without significant cardiovascular problems
should be cardiac monitored for a minimum of 24 hours
on a cardiac monitoring unit. Patients that have any
of the symptoms of cardiac toxicity such as sinus tachycardia over 140, arrhythmias, or block should be monitored for 72 hours beyond the time that the irregularities were reversed. All patients should be reviewed
by the psychiatry service to evaluate the potential for
further suicide and to evaluate the degree of depression.
Obviously follow up visits should be recommended to
determine residual effects of this acute toxic episode.
If the ingestion was in a child, careful determination
of the circumstances relating to the ingestion should
be made to rule out child abuse or poor home safety.

In summary, dealing with a tricyclic antidepressant
overdose is challenging since we are dealing with
various acute syndromes. The symptoms do not progress
linearly in one direction, i.e. excitation or depression, but rather are reflections of four stages of
pharmacodynamics. By utilizing this model of stages
it is easier to follow the course of the toxicity as
well as the success of the treatment regime. The
four stages are:

1. Delayed absorption → vagal block
2. Vagal block → catechol enhancement
3. Catechole enhancement → catechol depletion
4. Complete catechol depletion

The basic principles of tricyclic antedepressant
poison treatment are: prevent absorption, specific
antagonism, and nonspecific antagonism.

A final important aspect in dealing with these
toxicities is to attempt to influence the prescribing
habits of physicians regarding total size of the pre-
scription, close follow up of patient course during
therapy, rational of other drugs in combination with

tricyclics and lastly the accurate diagnosis of the patients underlying psychiatric state. Pediatricians should likewise be warned to caution parents of children receiving these agents.

TABLE 1

Coma Stage	Description of Stage
0	Verbally arousable, oriented X3
1	Noxious arousal, DTR +2 (deep tendon reflexes)
2	No arousal, DTR +1
3	No Arousal, no DTR
4	Above, plus cardiorespiratory deficiency

REFERENCES

1. Brashares ZA, Conley WR: Physostigmine in drug overdose. *Emergency Case Reports* 46-48, Jan-Feb 1975.

2. Brown TCK, Barker GA, Dunlop ME, et al: The use of sodium bicarbonate in the treatment of tricyclic antidepressant-induced arrhythmias. *Anaesthesia and Intensive Care* I:3:203-210, 1973.

3. Crocker J, Morton B: Tricyclic (antidepressant) drug toxicity. *Clin Toxicol* 2:4:397-402, 1969.

4. Duvoisin RC, Katz R: Reversal of central anti-cholinergic syndrome in man by physostigmine. *JAMA* 206:9:1963-1965, 1968.

5. Gard HD, Knapp I, Hanenson T, et al: Studies on the disposition of amitriptyline and other tricyclic antidepressant drugs in man as it relates to the management of the overdosed patient. *Advances in Biochem Pharmacol* 7:95-105, 1973.

6. Goel KM, Shanks RA: Amitriptyline and imipramine poisoning in children. *British Med J* I:261-263, 1974.

7. Jefferson JW: A review of the cardiovascular effects and toxicity of tricyclic antidepressants. *Psychosomatic Med* 37:2:160-179, 1975.

8. Newton RW: Physostigmine salicylate in the treatment of tricyclic antidepressant overdosage. *JAMA* 231:9:941-943, 1975.

9. Rumack BH: Anticholinergic poisoning:Treatment of 707 patients with physostigmine. Paper read at the *Amer Clin Toxicol Meeting,* August 12-16, 1974.

10. Rumack BH: Anticholinergic poisoning:Treatment with physostigmine. *Pediatrics* 52:3, 1973.

11. Slovis TL, Ott JE, Teitelbaum DT, Lipscomb W: psysostigmine Therapy in Acute Tricyclic Antidepressant Poisoning. *Clin Toxicol* 4:451-459, 1971.

12. Williams RB, Jr, Sherter C: Cardiac Complications of Tricyclic Antidepressant Therapy. *Annals of Internal Medicine* 74:395-398, 1971.

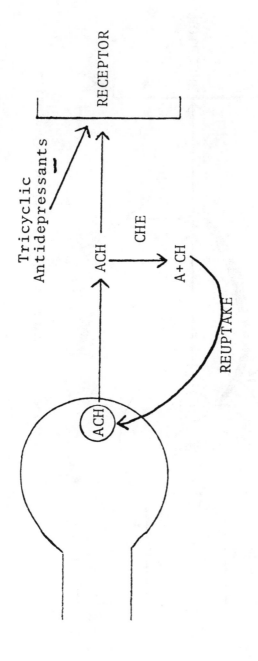

Figure 1. Anticholinergenic Action

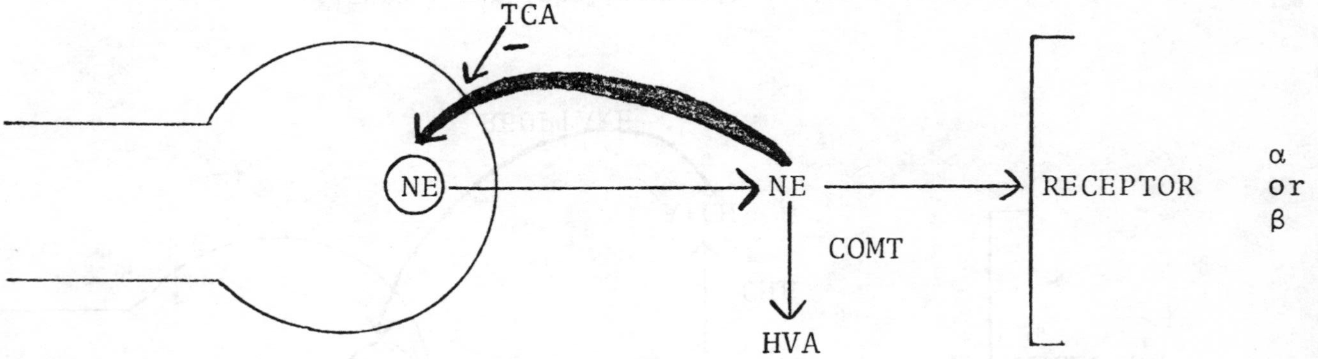

Figure 2. Enhanced α and β Receptor Stimulation

PHARMACOKINETIC OBSERVATIONS IN THE TREATMENT OF PHENCYCLIDINE POISONING. A PRELIMINARY REPORT

Alan K. Done, M.D.
Professor of Pediatrics and Pharmacology, Wayne State University School of Medicine, Detroit Director of Clinical Pharmacy and Toxicology, Children's Hospital of Michigan

Regine Aronow, M.D.
Director Poison Control Center, Children's Hospital of Michigan, Assistant Professor of Pediatrics at Wayne University School of Medicine

Joseph N. Miceli, Ph.D
Director, Clinical Pharmacology and Toxicology Laboratories at Children's Hospital of Michigan Assistant Professor of Pharmacology, Wayne State University School of Medicine

Dennis C.K. Lin
Battelle Columbus Laboratories, Detroit

ABSTRACT

Pharmacokinetic studies were performed in patients who had overdosed themselves with this currently popular "street" drug, with the aims of 1) elucidating the reasons for the characteristically prolonged and vacillating course of severe poisoning and 2) improving treatment. With presenting serum PCP levels of about 100-300 ng/ml (associated with coma), the serum half-life was in the range of 1 to 3 days. PCP levels in gastrointestinal drainage were high (as much as 4-6 x serum) and paralleled serum levels, suggesting pH-dependent GI recirculation. Peritoneal (dialysis) clearance, even with added albumin, was modest as compared with potential urinary excretion. Urinary excretion of PCP was markedly pH-dependent and exactly paralleled pH-partition coefficients: as expected from the drug's pKa of 8.5, acidification of the urine by administration of NH_4Cl caused a 10-fold

increase of clearance in a urine of pH 6.5 and more
than a 100-fold increase when the urine pH was 5.5 or
lower. Acidification was also associated with striking
clinical improvement. Superimposition of furosemide
diuresis (upon urine acidification) produced an addi-
tional almost doubling of PCP clearance.

PHENCYCLIDINE KINETICS

Phencyclidine 1-(Phenylcyclohexyl) piperidine (PCP),
was investigated as an analgesic-anesthetic agent, but
was discarded for human use because of severe dysphoric
effects, and for several years has been marketed only
as a sedative and tranquilizer for non-human primates.
It has recently emerged as one of the most important
drugs of abuse, beginning with its apparent "street"
introduction (as the "Peace Pill") in 1967 in San
Francisco (1), and is now controlled under the comprehensive Drug Abuse Prevention and Control Act of
1970. After a period of brief popularity, PCP fell
into disrepute as a "street" drug, but was commonly
misrepresented as other psychedelic compounds, as
tetrahydrocannabinol (THC), LSD, mescaline etc., and
in this manner became one of the drugs most commonly
encountered unexpectedly among intoxications from
abused drugs in major areas of the USA (2-6). Illic-
itly manufactured PCP appears now to be regaining
some popularity as an intended drug of abuse, in at
least the Detroit area.

PCP abuse has involved oral, parenteral and inha-
lational routes, and both one-time exploratory and
chronic intermittent or regular use. Effects of low
doses include disordered thought processes, distor-
tions of body image and proprioception, exaggerated
or disorganized responses to sensory input, flushing, diaphoresis, nystagmus, hallucinations and extreme agitation (7). At higher doses, coma, dystonia,
convulsions and sometimes hypertension, respiratory

depression and apnea may also occur (2,5,8), and the
electroencephalogram (EEG) is distinctively abnormal
(9,10); fatalities have been associated with status
epilepticus (2,13) and, in keeping with the known
sympathomimetic effects of PCP (12), with hypertensive
crisis (11).

The course of PCP poisoning is characterized by
extraordinarily prolonged symptoms among the most
severe cases, marked fluctuations in state of consciousness with abrupt awakening and unexplained re-
lapses, and persistence of PCP in urine for at least
several days in some cases (2,5,8,11,18). The scant
available pharmacokinetic data provide neither expla-
nations for such observations nor bases for treatment
of PCP intoxication. We had the opportunity to study
patients with severe PCP poisoning, employing a more
specific and sensitive quantitative method than here-
tofore has been available (14). This is a report of
the preliminary pharmacokinetic observations and some
resulting therapeutic recommendations.

SUBJECTS AND METHODS

The subjects of this study were three adolescent
males who were admitted to Children's Hospital of
Michigan after they overdosed themselves during
phencyclidine abuse. Clinical data and admission and
peak PCP blood-levels for these patients are recorded
in Table I. After becoming comatose at home, all
three briefly received treatment at another hospital
prior to transfer to Children's Hospital of Michigan,
and so all details of early course and treatment are
not available; the time of transfer corresponds to
the times of the admission PCP measurements noted in
Table I.

Patients 1 and 2 shared material chewed from a
putty-like, amorphous "cake", and patient 3 took
tablets, 15 of which were recovered with gastric

lavage about 16 hours post-ingestion. In each case the ingested material was from "underground" sources and apparently of illicit manufacture so that details of its compounding and composition are not available. However, samples both of the material actually ingested and of gastric contents were submitted to analysis in a gas chromatograph/mass spectrometer/computer system described elsewhere (6), and phencyclidine was identified as the sole major ingredient on the basis of mass spectral similarities to those published (15) for reference compounds.

Histories of prior drug-use experience were deemed not reliable: Patient 3 was known frequently to be involved in drug abuse and had had at least one previous overdosage episode, though it was uncertain whether or to what extent he had previously used PCP; Patients 1 and 2 were thought to have been, at most, only occasional experimenters with unspecified drug abuse, but allegedly not previously involving PCP.

For PCP measurements, blood specimens (from antecubital veins) and the entire bladder content of urine were obtained at the start of the study period; then quantitative 6-hour urine collections were made and blood specimens were obtained mid-way therein. Such sampling was intermittent in Patients 1 and 2 and continuous in Patient 3 throughout the study period. In Patients 2 and 3, the stomach was lavaged with 500 ml 0.9% saline at the time of admission and again at the start of the study period (Patient 3 was also lavaged previously at another hospital within a few hours after PCP ingestion); lavage was not performed here in Patient 1 (who was admitted 2 1/2 days post-ingestion), but had been performed at another hospital within a few hours after PCP ingestion. The nasogastric lavage tube was left in place in Patients 2 and 3 and continuous drainage was collected quantitatively in 6-hour aliquots which were timed to coincide with the urine collections. The gastric drainage volumes ranged from 150 to 432 ml and averaged 270 ml (45 ml per hour). Measurements of pH were made in urine and gastric fluid with a Beckman (Model 3550) pH meter and in arterial blood with an Instrumentation Laboratories Model 113 electrometer using a Severinghaus pH electrode.

After observations in Patients 1 and 2 suggested enhanced PCP excretion in acid urine (vide infra), efforts to acidify the urine of Patient 3 were undertaken: ammonium chloride, 2 g dissolved in 60 ml 0.9% saline, was introduced through a separate nasogastric tube at the start of each 6-hour drainage period, the tube was flushed through with a similar volume of saline, and the tube for collection of gastric secretions was clamped for two hours before drainage was resumed. Ascorbic acid, 1 g, was added to each 6-hour intravenous infusion.

In the absence of information about the dialyzability of PCP and the effect of pH on its urinary excretion, peritoneal dialysis was employed in Patient 2 because of his serious condition and in order to evaluate effectiveness of the procedure and the partitioning of PCP between blood and peritoneal fluid. Conventional peritoneal dialysis fluid containing 1.5% glucose* with the addition of 3 mEq KCL and 500 u heparin per liter was infused into the peritoneal cavity in volumes usually of 1500 ml, then drained, each hour. In two instances, human serum albumin was added in a concentration of 5% to determine the influence of protein on PCP partitioning.

Specimens were frozen until analyzed for PCP concentrations. Quantification of PCP in body fluids was by the gas chromatographic/chemical ionization mass

---

*Dianeal (R), Travenol

spectrometric method of Lin, et al (14). Measurements
were confined to the free, unchanged compound; specifically, there was no attempt to measure its known hy-
droxylated metabolities which are found as glucuronides
in urine (PCP itself is not so conjugated)(14,16,17).
PCP clearances via urinary excretion, gastric drainage
and peritoneal dialysis were calculated by: [PCP] x
volume/minutes x [PCP]$_{serum}$.

RESULTS

The clinical course of patients 2 and 3 is detailed
in Figure 1 in relation to the time-course of serum
PCP concentrations and the therapeutic procedures that
were instituted. Despite substantial differences in
the rate of decline of serum PCP (serum half-live
about 3.7 vs 1 day in these two subjects), there was
a striking similarity in the relation of serum PCP
level to state of consciousness. Both patients were
consistently comatose with levels above about 125
ng/ml, but could be aroused at least intermittently
(designated "semi-coma") after the level had dropped
below about 90 ng/ml. Frank disorientation was present
until the levels dropped to below about 25 ng/ml.

Electroencephalograms were too few to establish a
relationship, but levels above about 60 ng/ml were
associated with both delta rhythm and dysrhythmia.
The delta rhythm disappeared first at roughly the same
blood level as the disorientation, and normalcy of EEG
probably did not occur until the level was at 20 ng/ml
or even lower. Patient 3, despite a higher level of
PCP in serum had none of the convulsions exhibited
frequently by patient 2 during the first three days,
but an explanation for this difference could not be
ascertained.

Reasons for the difference in rate of decline of
serum PCP concentrations likewise were not suggested

by our data. Despite repeated gestric lavage and continuous gastric drainage, both patients had brief rises
in serum PCP levels, but thereafter the levels declined
in an approximately first-order fashion, except for the
step-wise fluctuations shown by patient 2. The latter's
occasional plateaus may have been attributable to certain
therapeutic procedures, since one followed immediately
upon discontinuance of peritoneal dialysis, and another
occurred when gastric drainage was stopped. Patient 3
also had a minor rise in serum PCP and a slower decline
when gastric drainage was stopped. Although urine acidification with ammonium chloride in patient 3 greatly
increased PCP excretion (vide infra), it can be seen in
Figure I that the serum level continued to decline at
approximately the same rate as previously and its relationship to the clinical course remained unaltered. The
difference in rate of PCP elimination from sera of the
two subjects was not attributable to urine output, since
the rate was 89 ml/M^2/hr in patient 2 and 62 ml/M^2/hr
in patient 3. The two patients also had comparable
volumes of gastric drainage. The concentration of PCP
in their urine and gastric drainage bore similar relationships to pH, but patient 2 had less acidic excretion
of both fluids, as will become evident from the clearance
data.

Concentration curves of PCP in serum and gastric
drainage were strikingly parallel, with the latter
being about 30 to 50 times higher (Figure 2). Even
minor shifts in the concentration curves were parallel
in these two fluids, with serum reflecting a change
slightly later than the gastric fluid, and the rate
of decline was the same in the two fluids (half-life =
0.9 d in patient 3: the serum concentration half-life
in this individual was 1.1 d after discontinuance of
gastric drainage). The PCP concentration in urine
fluctuated tremendously with changes in pH (vide infra),
but was almost invariably much higher than that in
serum.

The cumulative excretion data of Figure 2 suggest
that the total PCP elimination via these two routes in
patient 3 over the course of study was about 31 mg:
just over 16 mg in 3 days by the gastric route, and
nearly 15 mg by urinary excretion in 6 days (almost
all of this occurring in the first 4 days). The cumulative urinary excretion showed a tendency to plateau
when the urine pH was above about 6 and to accelerate
when it was more acidic.

Figure 3 presents data concerning the relationship
of pH to the partitioning of PCP between serum and
various body fluids, including urine, gastric and peritoneal fluid. The concentration gradient favoring
urine over serum increased progressively with increasing
acidity, such that urines with pH in the range of 4.5
had PCP concentrations nearly 200-times those of serum.
The concentrations in peritoneal fluid were slightly
lower than those in serum, and had a lower concentration
ration with serum than did urines at similar pH. While
gastric fluids routinely had much higher concentrations
than serum, and tended perhaps to be highest with greatest acidity, they fell well below the pH-dependent partitioning exhibited by urine. The data of Figure 3
suggest that ammonium chloride administration influenced
PCP concentration in urine and GI drainage only insofar
as it affected pH, at least of urine.

To explore further the mechanism of the pH effect on
urinary PCP, the ratio of urine to serum PCP concentration was plotted against urine pH in Figure 4. With
decreasing urine pH, at least in the range of pH 7.5
to 5.5, there was a striking similarity between the
actual observations and the ratio predicted on the
basis of pH effects on ionization of PCP, assuming a
plasma pH of 7.4 and a pK_a of 8.5* for PCP. With

---

*Documentation could not be found for the frequently
quoted (or any other) pK_a of about 8.5 for PCP. Our
studies thusfar indicate at least that the partition
coefficient for PCP between water and chloroform is
one at a pH of about 8.5, and the data of Figure 4
are consistent with a pK_a of 8.5.

urines of pH less than 5.5 there may be a lag in the
urine/serum relationship. There were too few data
points to determine whether ammonium chloride administration perhaps tilted the curve downward at low pH and
upward at high pH, but certainly there was no great
effect of ammonium chloride except as it altered urine
pH.

The relationship of renal clearance of PCP to urine
pH, urine volume and certain clinical events is illus-
trated for one patient in Figure 5. In this individual
(patient 3) the administration of ammonium chloride via
nasogastric tube produced no measurable decline in blood
pH and only a minor and transient serum chloride excess.
It resulted, however, in a marked fall in urine pH to
levels near 4.5, with a gradual rise after its discontinuance. The decline in urine pH was associated with
a greatly increased PCP clearance rate, rivaled only
by ones observed initially and subsequently during
periods of spontaneously acidic urine and comparatively
marked diuresis. The enhanced PCP clearance during
ammonium chloride administration occurred despite an
actual decline in urine volume, probably the result of
inadequate fluid administration.

While increased urine volume appeared to enhance further the augmenting effect of acidification on PCP
clearance, it appeared to have little effect when the
urine was not acidified: for example, the diuresis
that occurred around the two and the 5½ to 7 day periods,
when the urine was relatively alkaline, did not produce
an increment in PCP clearance. The extent to which
forced diuresis might have furthered PCP elimination
was not determined in this study.

Figure 5 compares the clearance of PCP by the various
modalities studied. The highest clearances were obtained
with acidic urine. Peritoneal dialysis was relatively
ineffective; in fact was no more efficient than excretion even in relatively alkaline urine, and far less

efficient than excretion in an acid urine. The inclusion of albumin in the dialysis fluid produced only a minor improvement that still did not rival optimal urinary excretion. Gastric drainage, however, resulted in clearance of as much PCP as all but the most acidic urines. Except for the one 500 ml lavage of the stomach, we unfortunately did not determine whether a more effective gastric dialysis could have been obtained by promoting larger volumes and/or by introducing acidic solutions to wash the stomach.

DISCUSSION

In the human, phencyclidine metabolism involves formation of mono-hydroxylated derivatives (14,16,17), apparently two in number (14), which are then excreted in the urine. The free drug is also extensively excreted in urine. Metabolites have not been demonstrated in the blood, and metabolities in the urine are present entirely as glucuronides (14). The analytical method used in this study measures only unchanged phencyclidine; consequently, the results are relevant only to kinetics of the parent compound. While this serves the purposes of explaining the clinical course of PCP poisoning and providing possible bases for its treatment, the approach does not define the overall fate of phencyclidine in human intoxication. Such studies are currently underway.

The protracted time-course of serum PCP, reflected in half-life values of one to nearly four days in our patients with severe phencyclidine poisoning are in keeping with the prolonged course described by others (2,5,8,11,18). Our data suggest that there is considerable secretion of PCP into the stomach; indeed, levels in acidic gastric secretions were 30 to 50 times higher than in serum, most likely because of pH-dependent ion-trapping of this weak base. This observation has practical importance not only in terms of the therapeutic considerations noted below, but also because it indicates that the presence of high concentrations of PCP in gastric content does not at all

suggest oral ingestion, a fact that can be of considerable forensic interest. Of importance to the course
of PCP poisoning is the likelihood that PCP secreted
into the stomach may become non-ionized in its passage
through more alkaline areas of the intestional tract,
and therefore eligible for reabsorption, thus prolong-
ing the course.

The urinary excretion of unchanged PCP has a pattern
of pH-dependence that with some reservations,* suggests
a pure ionization effect, again with ion-trapping in
the acidic urine. At the very high urine-to-serum concentration ratios obtained with very acidic urines,
there was some suggestion that the concentration gradients actually attained fell somewhat below those
theoretically possible, though there was generally
good agreement between observed and predicted gradients. In current studies, using therapy more effective
in promoting renal blood flow and function, we are
attempting to determine whether it is possible to
achieve the maximally predictable urine-to-serum concentration gradient (e.g., circa 700 x at urine pH =
4.5 and blood pH = 7.4).

The failure of gastric secretions even to approach
concentration gradients with serum of the magnitude
predicted by ionization theory is not explained by
our data, but there is ample precedent for this observation (19). It is possible that this reflects limited delivery of drug to the gastric mucosa via the
circulation. In fact, the present data demonstrate

---

*If the pK_a for PCP is, in fact, about 8.5. We would
not propose, however, that the data of Figure 4 be accepted simultaneously as evidence for a pK_a of about
8.5 as well as a pure ionization effect. The latter
conclusion presumes the former and would require mod-
ification if a significantly different pK_a were proved.

a limiting concentration ratio which is very close to
the one of 40 described by Brodie from dog experiments
employing aniline (20). The effective concentration
gradient for diffusion of a base having a much higher
pK_a than the pH of plasma may be reduced because a
major fraction of the circulating drug would be ionized,
but such a factor should have affected partitioning
between serum and gastric fluid or urine alike and
would not account for the differences (depicted in
Figure 3) between these two fluids in the relationship
of the concentration gradients to pH.

PCP concentration in peritoneal dialysis fluid ap-
proached those in serum, the ratios being just below
those achieved in urine at similar pH. The data suggest the possibility that a higher gradient between
peritoneal fluid and serum might have been achieved
using a fluid of more acidic pH, but whether tolerable
acidification of such fluid would produce PCP removal
increments that would rival those achievable by urine
acidification and/or gastric drainage remains to be
determined.

The possibility that differences in PCP metabolism
or distribution accounted for the striking inter-
patient differences in rate of removal of PCP from
circulation noted in our subjects is currently being
explored. During urine acidification with ammonium
chloride and ascorbic acid, Patient 3 excreted much
larger quantities of PCP in the urine than did the
other subjects, but he had a more rapid fall in serum
PCP concentrations both before and after the period of
acidification than did the other subjects. Whether
prior exposure to PCP was involved in these subjects
and could have altered PCP elimination is unclear.
Patient 3 was, however, more likely than the others
to have had previous PCP use and also had the fastest
decline of serum PCP. The relationship of prior PCP
use to metabolism and/or excretion of the drug is
being explored.

The treatment of phencyclidine poisoning has been entirely symptomatic and supportive, and unsatisfactory at best. The observations of this report provide rationale for improved approaches to therapy. While urine acidification has been shown to promote the urinary excretion of a variety of weak bases, the increment in PCP excretion achieved thereby was extraordinary, if not unparalleled.

What constitutes adequate acidification of the urine in cases of severe phencyclidine poisoning is a matter of judgement that must take the urgency of the situation into account. However, the data of Figure 3 suggest that the effectiveness does not begin to rise strikingly until the urine pH is reduced at least to about 5.5, and climbs dramatically when the pH drops below 5.0. The ability to reach maximum urine-to-plasma concentration gradients through ion-trapping may be compromised by factors other than pH per se, but the possibility exists that this restriction could be overcome by enhancing renal blood flow and/or function. The present data certainly suggest the desirability of combining urine acidification with diuresis.

Continuous gastric drainage also appears to be an important therapuetic procedure. It seems possible that its effectiveness could be enhanced still further by perfusing the stomach with modest volumes of exogenous fluid, particularly if the latter was itself of sufficiently low pH. Using, for example, a solution of hydrochloric acid at pH of about 2 might have the additional advantage of preventing the alkalosis that is possible with prolonged drainage and/or in young children.

Diazepam has been used extensively to combat the seizures or excitement of phencyclidine poisoning, and we have no real evidence to condemn its use in this situation. However, the observation that its frequent administration was peculiar to our patient

who had the longest serum half-life for PCP cause us
to advise the avoidance at least of prolonged or repeated use until this question is resolved.

SUMMARY

Preliminary pharmacokinetic studies in three patients
overdosed during phencyclidine (PCP) abuse suggest that
the prolonged course of severe PCP poisoning occurs
pari passu with a slow decline in serum concentration
of PCP (half-life one to nearly four days). PCP was
found to be concentrated markedly in gastric secretions
and in acid urines relative to serum, probably on the
basis of ion-trapping. While there were unidentified
constraints on the augmenting effects of acidity on
PCP partitioning between serum and gastric fluid, this
gastrointestinal recirculation of PCP was appreciable
and probably contributes to the persistence of PCP in
the body and to the prolonged course of severe PCP
poisoning. Peritoneal dialysis, even with added
albumin, was relatively ineffective, removing much
less PCP than was achievable by urine acidification.
Diuresis appeared to augment PCP excretions still further in acidic urine, but had little effect when the
urine was alkaline. Improved therapeutic approaches
to phencyclidine poisoning suggested by these data
include promotion of diuresis after acidification of
the urine to pH 5.0 or lower, and continuous gastric
drainage and/or gastric dialysis.

REFERENCES

1. Meyers RH, Rose AJ, Smith DE: Incidents involving the Haight-Ashbury population and some uncom-
monly used drugs. *J Psychedelic Drugs* 1:139-146,
1967-1968.

2. Burns RS, Lerner SE, Corrado R, et al: Phen-
cyclidine--states of acute intoxication and fatalities.
West J Med 123:345-49, 1975.

3. Rainey JM, Crowder MK: Prevalence of phencyclidine in street drug preparations. *N Engl J Med*
290:466-467, 1974.

4. Hart JB, McChesney JC, Grief M, et al: Composition of illicit drugs and use of drug analysis in
abuse abatement. *J Psychedelic Drugs* 5:(I)83-88,
1972.

5. Liden CB, Lovejoy FH, Costello CE: Phencyclidine: Nine cases of poisoning. *JAMA* 234:513-516,
1975.

6. Horwitz JP, Hills EB, Andrejewski D, et al:
Adjunct hospital emergency toxicology service: A model
for a metropolitan area. *JAMA* 235:1708-1712, 1976.

7. Domino EF: Neurobiology of phencyclidine
(sernyl): A drug with unusual spectrum of pharmacology
activity. *Int Rev Neurobiol* 6:303-347, 1964.

8. Tong TG, Benowitz NL, Becker CE, et al: Phencyclidine poisoning. *JAMA* 234:512-513, 1975.

9. Meyer JS, Griefenstein F, DeVault M: A new
drug causing symptoms of sensory deprivation: neurological, electroencephalographic and pharmacological
effects of sernyl. *J Nerv Ment Dis* 129:54-61, 1959.

10. Rodin EA, Luby ED, Meyer JS: Electroencephalographic findings associated with sernyl infusion. *Electroencephalography & Clin Neurophys J* 11:796-798, 1959.

11. Eastman JW, Cohen SN: Hypertensive crisis and death associated with phencyclidine poisoning. *JAMA* 231:1270-1270-1271, 1975.

12. Chen G, Easor CR, Russell D, et al: The pharmacology of 1-(1-phenylcyclohexyl) piperidine HCL. *J Pharmacol Exp Ther* 127:241-250, 1959.

13. Kessler GF, Demers LM, Berlin C, et al: Phencyclidine and fatal status epilepticus. *N Engl J Med* 291:979, 1974.

14. Lin DCK, Fentiman AF, Foltz RL, et al: Quantification of phencyclidine in body fluids by gas chromatography chemical ionization mass spectrometry and identification of two metabolites. *Biomed Mass Spectrom* 2:206-214, 1975.

15. Biemann K (ed): *Mass Spectra of Drugs*. Cambridge, Massachusetts, MIT Department of Chemistry, 1971.

16. Ober RE, Gwynn GW, Chang T, et al: Metabolism of 1-(1-phenylcyclohexyl) piperidine (sernyl). *Fed Proc* 22:539, 1963.

17. Lin DCK, Foltz RL, Done AK, et al: Mass spectrometric analysis of phencyclidine in body fluids of intoxicated patients, in *Proceedings of an International Symposium on Quantitative Mass Spectrometry in Life Sciences*. Gent, Belgium, 1976.

18. Gupta RC, Lu I, Oei GL, et al: Determination of phencyclidine (PCP) in urine and illicit street drug samples. *Clin Toxicol* 8:611-621, 1975.

19.   Goldstein A, Aronow L, Kalman SM: *Principles of Drug Action: The basis of pharmacology, ed 2.* New York, John Wiley & Sons, 1974.

20.   Brodie BB, Hogben AM: Some physico-chemical factors in drug action.   *J Pharm & Pharmacol* 9:345-380, 1957.

TABLE I

PATIENT DATA

Patient	Age (Yrs/Mos)	Weight (Kg)	Serum PCP, ng/ml (and interval post-ingestion) t admission+	peak measured	Clinical manifestations	Duration (from time of ingestion)	Treatment*
1 (RM)	13/11	40	74 (2.5da)	Same	coma, hypertonus hallucinations, nystagmus disorient., hyperacusis electroencephalographic abnorm.: delta rhythm dysrhythmia	4 hr 8 hr 3- 4 da 7- 9 da 9+da	none
2 (TS)	14/0	53	100 (0.5da)	210(1.0&2.2da)	coma convulsions, hypertonus, laryngospasm hallucinations, agitation disorientation electroencephalographic abnorm.: delta rhythm dysrhythmia	4 da 3 da 10 da 15 da 8- 10 da 10- 14 da	Gastric drainage Peritoneal dialysis Diazepam (Frequent) Methicillin
3 (GC)	18/0	45	264 (1.8da)	329(2.3 da)	coma, hypertonus agitation disorientation electroencephalographic abnorm.: delta rhythm dysrythmia	2½da 3 da 5 da 3- 8 da 8+da	Gastric drainage NH4Cl Ascorbate (Diazepam, once only on day 2) (Furosemide, 40 mg IV at day 1.3)

*In addition to the supportive care, gastric lavage, and intravenous fluids given to all three

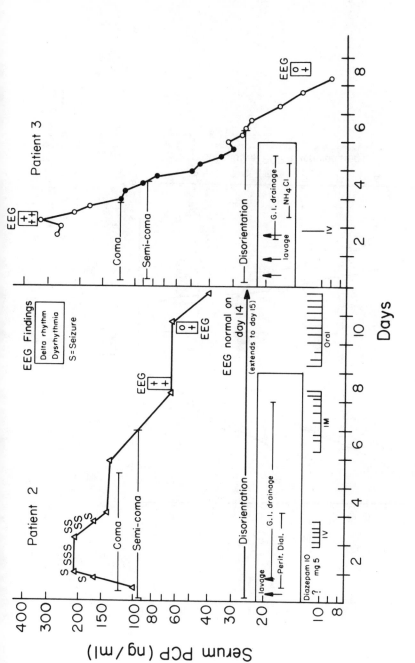

Figure 1. Time-course of serum [PCP] in relation to clinical findings and procedures in Patients 2 and 3. Solid points are for periods of maximum ammonium chloride-induced acidity (pH < 5.5) of urine.

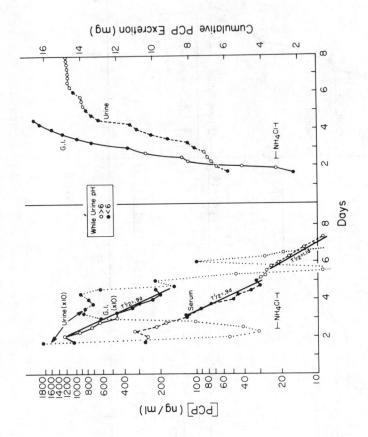

Figure 2. Correlation of [PCP] in serum, urine and gastric drainage (left) and cumulative urinary and gastric secretions of PCP (right) in Patient3. Note that urine and gastric (G.I.) concentrations were 10x higher than shown in the left-hand figure.

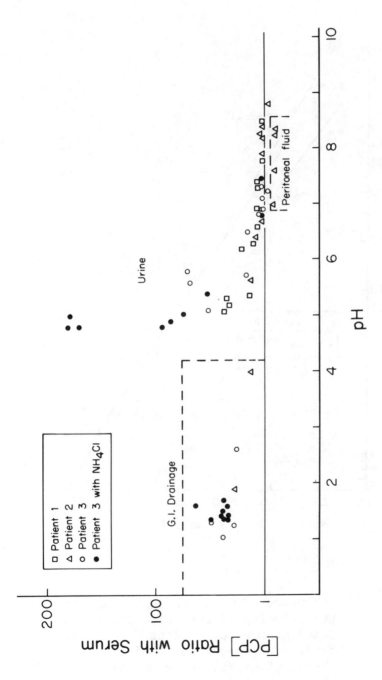

Figure 3. pH and the ratio of [PCP] in body fluids and serum.

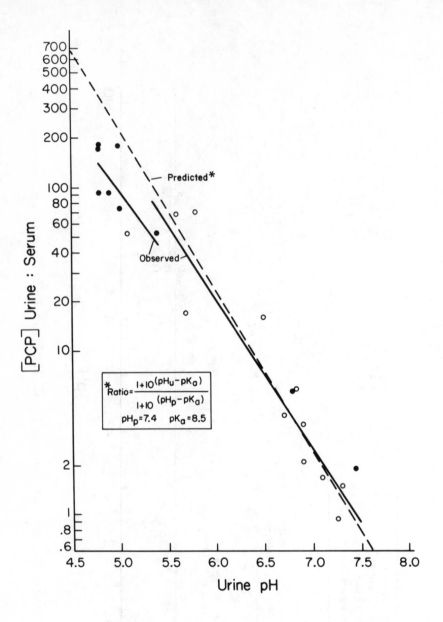

Figure 4. Influence of urine pH on the urine: serum partitioning of PCP, as observed in Patient 3 and as predicted (dotted line) on the basis of pH-dependant ionization using a plasma pH of 7.4 and a pK_a of 8.5 for PCP. (Solid points are for the period of NH_4CL administration).

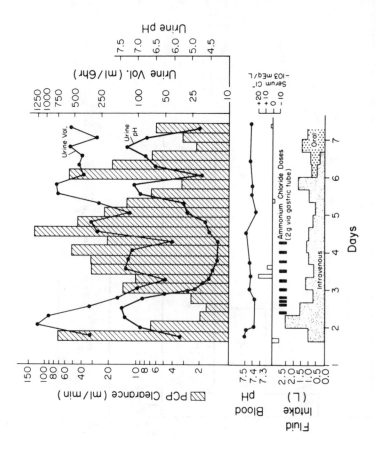

Figure 5. Renal clearance of PCP in relation to urine pH, urine volume and clinical events in Patient 3.

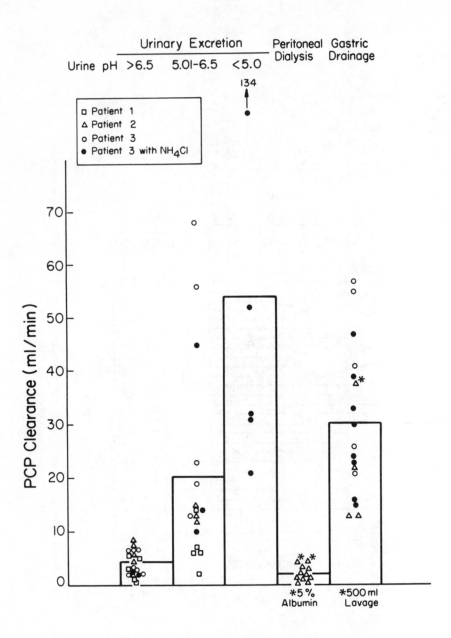

Figure 6. Comparative PCP clearance (ml serum per minute) via urinary excretion at various pH's, peritoneal dialysis, and gastric drainage.

SERUM CONCENTRATION STUDIES DURING HEMODIALYSIS IN A
PATIENT WITH SEVERE METHANOL INTOXICATION *

Anthony S. Manoguerra, Pharm.D.
Director, Hennepin County Poison Control Center,
  Minneapolis
Assistant Professor of Pharmacy, University of
  Minnesota

Robert J. Cipolle, Pharm.D.
Staff member, St. Paul Ramsey Hospital and Medical
  Center, St. Paul
Instructor in Pharmacy, University of Minnesota

Darwin E. Zaske, Pharm.D.
Staff member, St. Paul Ramsey Hospital and Medical
  Center, St. Paul
Assistant Professor of Pharmacology, University of
  Minnesota

Sally M. Ehlers, M.D.
Staff member, Section of Nephrology, St. Paul Ramsey
  Hospital and Medical Center, St. Paul

ABSTRACT

   The patient was a 50-year old white male admitted to
the hospital following ingestion of an unknown quantity
of Heet Gasline Antifreeze over the previous 48 hours.
The product contains 94.5% methanol, 4% isopropanol
and 1.5% antioxidants. On admission, the patient was
alert and fully oriented with complaints of blurred

---

*The authors would like to express their appreciation
to Ronald Sawchuck, Ph.D., Assistant Professor of
Pharmacokinetics at the University of Minnesota
College of Pharmacy for his assistance in the development of the dosing schedules.

*vision. Blood gases showed marked acidosis and a
methanol level was 280 mg%. Hemodialysis was instituted and the pharmacokinetics of methanol during dialysis
was studied. The ethanol levels achieved with a 1 mg/kg
oral loading dose and subsequent maintenance doses,
both during dialysis and post dialysis, were also studied.
Two ophthalmologic examinations after dialysis showed
no visual impairment.*

We recently had the opportunity to treat a case of
severe methanol poisoning using hemodialysis and concurrent oral administration of ethanol. We monitored
the effectiveness of dialysis by performing serial
serum methanol determinations. Ethanol therapy was
performed using suggested dosages from the literature,
which produced suboptimal serum ethanol levels during
dialysis and potentially toxic levels post-dialysis.
We would, therefore, like to report the case, discuss
the results of serum studies and suggest a more accurate dosing schedule based on pharmacokinetic principles
and calculations.

The patient was a 50 year old male inventor at 3M
Company. He presented to the emergency department at
St. Paul - Ramsey Hospital with a history of ingesting
an unknown quantity of Heet Gasline Antifreeze, which
contains 94.5% methanol, 4% isopropanol and 1.5% antioxidants. The patient stated that he consumed an eight
ounce can of Heet over the previous 48 hours, but his
history was considered to be unreliable. When his wife
discovered what he had done, she immediately brought him
to the hospital, although the patient felt it was unnecessary. The patient stated that he ingested the
Heet to "see what it would do".

On arrival, the patient's subjective complaints were
nausea and blurred vision in his central fields. Ob-
jectively, he was a normal appearing adult male, mildly
lethargic, with shallow rapid respirations. His labora-

tory data showed a sodium of 139 meq/L, potassium
4.8 meq/L, carbon dioxide less than 10 meq/L, chloride
100 meq/L., blood urea nitrogen 14 mg/100 ml., blood
gases: pH 7.16, pO_2 125 mm Hg., pCO_2 14 mm Hg., bicarbonate 4.8 meq/L., and a methanol level of 282 mg%.
His body weight was 80 kg.

Intravenous fluids were started and the patient was
given 100 meq of sodium bicarbonate and was admitted
to the ward. The housestaff alerted the clinical
pharmacy service who then contacted the Hennepin County
Poison Control Center for consultation. It was decided to begin ethanol therapy and hemodialysis. The
patient was moved to the dialysis unit, sheldon cathe-
ters were placed and hemodialysis was begun. Concurrently, ethanol therapy was begun in the form of
Cabin Still 80 Proof Whiskey by the oral route.

He was given six ounces of whiskey orally over 30
minutes as a loading dose followed by a maintenance
dose of three ounces every two hours. He was dialyzed
for five hours at the end of which his methanol level
was 90 mg%. During dialysis he required an additional
250 meq of sodium bicarbonate to correct acidosis.
Ethanol therapy was continued for 36 hours after
dialysis was terminated. It was stopped because the
patient was experiencing increasing lethargy and disorientation.

On the patient's fourth hospital day, he was evaluated by the psychiatrists and was transferred to their
service because of apparent suicidal tendencies. He
was examined by the opthalmology service prior to the
transfer and several days later and they reported no
visual abnormalities. The patient is currently under-
going psychotherapy with no residual medical problems.

A review of the literature has revealed that this
case had the highest serum methanol level associated
with complete recovery reported in the literature.

All other patients with levels in this range either
died or were blinded by the ingestion. We feel that
this case further confirms the effectiveness of concurrent hemodialysis and ethanol therapy in methanol
poisoning.

Hemodialysis, as has been reported by other authors,
was extremely effective at removing methanol from this
patient. Assuming that adequate ethanol was present
to inhibit the hepatic elimination pathways of methanol,
dialysis was the sole route of elimination. Figure 1
shows the methanol levels reported on this patient
during treatment. Dialysis removed the methanol with
a half-life of 3.25 hours. Dialysis was stopped after
five hours leaving a methanol level of 90 mg%. In
retrospect a ten or twelve hour dialysis run should
have been performed which would have resulted in a
methanol level of less than 20 mg%.

The ethanol given to this patient resulted in the
ethanol levels shown in Figure 2. It is interesting
to note that this dosage of ethanol during dialysis
resulted in levels lower than the suggested level of
100 mg% that should be maintained. When dialysis was
stopped, the ethanol levels rose rapidly up to 240 mg%
at which time the ethanol was terminated.

We based our dosage of ethanol on several widely
used literature sources. This information is summarized in Table 1. Because of the extreme variation in
suggested doses, we chose the doses that we gave on a
somewhat empiric basis, using the 1ml/kg. of 100%
ethanol as a starting point. This dosage resulted in
levels that could have been less than optimal during
dialysis and post-dialysis levels that could have
produced severe ethanol toxicity.

We have, therefore, made some calculations based
on new data that was recently published on ethanol
kinetics and also on some data taken from this patient.

The elimination kinetics of ethanol are commonly referred to as zero order in nature, or independent of
the blood concentration. Wagner (1) has recently
published data that shows that ethanol does not follow
zero kinetics but actually follows Michaelis-Menten
kinetics, or so-called dose dependent kinetics.

Following are the calculations that we made which
provide a close approximation of the loading and
maintenance doses of ethanol needed both during
dialysis and when dialysis is not being used. We
have not had the opportunity to try this data on an
intoxicated patient as yet.

To calculate a loading dose of ethanol to develop
a serum level of 100 mg%:

$$\text{Dose} = Cp_O \times Vd$$
$$= 100 \text{ mg}/100 \text{ ml} \times 0.6 \text{ L/kg.}$$
$$= 0.6 \text{ Gm/Kg.}$$

where Cp_O is the peak serum concentration and Vd
is the volume of distribution.

The value for Vd that we used was derived from a
study of 23 patients given varying doses of ethanol (2).

To calculate a maintenance dose to maintain a level
of 100 mg% ethanol.

$$K_O = \frac{VM \ S}{Km + S} \quad \text{(Michaelis - Menten Equation)}$$

where K_O is the infusion or absorption rate,
assuming intravenous infusion or rapid oral
absorption, S is the serum concentration to
be maintained, Vm is the maximal elimination
rate and Km is the Michaelis constant.
Wagner (1) has determined the Km and Vm values

for ethanol as Vm:124 mg/kg hr and Km: 138 mg/L.

Therefore:

$$K_o = \frac{124 \text{ mg/kg hr} \times 100 \text{ mg/100 ml}}{138 \text{ mg/L} + 100 \text{ mg/ 100 ml.}}$$

$$K_o = 109 \text{ mg/kg hr}$$

Using this patient as an example: (Weight 80 kg)
To achieve a level of 100 mg% requires

Loading dose = 0.6 Gm/Kg x 80 kg.

= 48.0 Gm.

Using 80 Proof Ethanol = 40% $^V/_V$ = 31.7 Gm/100 ml.

$$\frac{48.0 \text{ Gm.}}{31.7 \text{ Gm/100 ml}} = 151 \text{ ml. of 80 proof whiskey.}$$

As the specific gravity of ethanol changes with the concentration of ethanol, it is important to consider this change in the calculations. For example, 40% ethanol by volume (80 proof) has 31.7 Gms/100 ml, whereas, 50% ethanol by volume (100 proof) has 39.7 Gms/100 ml.

To maintain a level of 100 mg% following a loading dose when the patient is not being dialyzed:

$$K_o = 109 \text{ mg/kg hr} \times 80 \text{ kg} = 8.72 \text{ Gms/hr}$$
Using 40% ethanol, K_o = 27.5 ml/hr.

To maintain a level of 100 mg% when the patient is being dialyzed:

$$K_D = K_o + DS \quad \text{where:} \quad K_D = \text{rate of administration during dialysis}$$
$$D = \text{dialysance}$$

According to the literature (3), the dialysance of ethanol and methanol in a given patient during a given dialysis run are the same. We therefore, calculated the dialysance of ethanol by calculating the dialysance of methanol using the data from this patient.

$$D = \frac{0.693 \ (Vd)}{t_{\frac{1}{2}}}$$
$$= \frac{0.693 \ (0.6 \ L/kg)}{3.25 \ hrs.}$$
$$= 0.128 \ L/kg \ hr.$$

Therefore,

$$K_D = 109 \ mg/kg \ hr + 128 \ ml/kg \ hr \ (100 \ mg/100 \ ml.)$$
$$= 109 \ mg/kg \ hr + 128 \ mg/kg \ hr$$
$$= 237 \ mg/kg \ hr.$$

For this patient:

$$K_D = 237 \ mg/kg \ hr \times 80 \ kg$$
$$= 18960 \ mg/hr.$$
$$= 59.8 \ ml/hr \ of \ 40\% \ ethanol.$$

Using these calculations, this patient should have received a five ounce loading dose of 80 proof ethanol followed by a maintenance dose of two ounces per hour during dialysis and one ounce per hour post-dialysis.

Several authors in the literature also suggest the use of a 5% ethanol solution intravenously if the patient cannot take oral ethanol. Using these calculations an 80Kg person would require a loading dose

of 1.2 liters and a maintenance dose of 693 ml/hr for
a total of almost 18 liters per day. This quantity of
fluid is not a realistic amount to give any patient
and therefore, 5% ethanol solutions intravenously
cannot be used.

In summary, ethanol therapy can be given according
to pharmacokinetic calculations to maintain a level
of 100 mg% both during dialysis and post-dialysis.
The equations necessary to calculate the required
dose are:

Loading dose = 0.6 Gm/kg.
Maintenance dose = 109 mg/kg hr.
Maintenance dose while being dialyzed = 237
mg/kg hr.

The dose calculated during dialysis will be an approximation that may vary according to the dialysis machine
used and the flow rate through the machine. However,
this calculation will place the dose near the 100%
level where it can be further adjusted based on
actual ethanol levels achieved.

TABLE 1

Suggested Ethanol Doses from the Literature

1. Gosselin [4] - 50% ethanol in a dose of 1 oz.
    every 3-4 hours.

2. Arena [5] - 45% ethanol in a dose of 3-4 oz.
    every 4 hours. In severe cases give 5% ethanol
    intravenously.

3. Poisindex [8] - 1cc/kg of 100% ethanol or 2cc/kg
    of 50% ethanol.

4. Matthew [6] - 50% ethanol as a loading dose of
    1 ml/kg followed by 0.5 ml/kg every 2 hours.

5. National Clearinghouse [7] - 0.75 Gm/kg loading
    dose followed by 0.5 Gms/kg every four hours.
    In severe cases give 5% ethanol intravenously.

REFERENCES

1. Wagner JG, Wilkinson PK, Sedman AJ, et al: Elimination of alcohol from human blood. *J Pharm Sci* 65:152-154, 1967.

2. Unpublished data from St. Paul Ramsey Hospital.

3. Knepshield JH, Schreiner GE, Lowenthal DT, et al: Dialysis of poisons and drugs. *Trans Amer Soc Artif Int Organs* 19:590-633, 1973.

4. Gosselin RE, Hodge HC, Smith RP, et al: *Clinical Toxicology of Commercial Products, ed 4*. Baltimore, Williams and Wilkins, 1976.

5. Arena JM: *Poisoning, ed 3*. Springfield, Charles Thomas, 1974.

6. Mathew H, Lawson AAH: *Treatment of Common Acute Poisonings*. Edinburgh, Churchill Livingstone, 1975.

7. *National Clearinghouse Cards*. Bethesda, distributed by the National Clearinghouse for Poison Control Centers, Food & Drug Administration.

8. *Poisindex*. Produced by the Micromedex Company in association with the Rocky Mountain Poison Center.

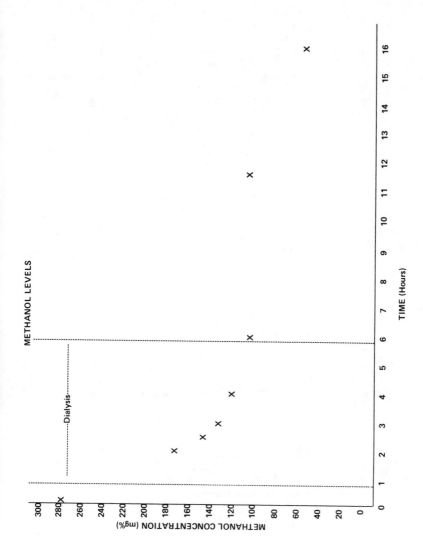

Figure 1. Methanol Concentration v. Time

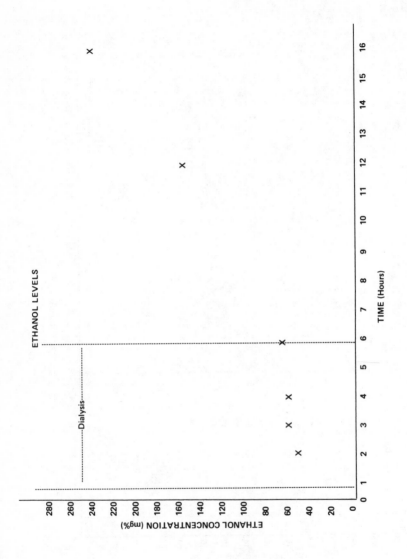

Figure 2. Ethanol Concentration v. Time

ACUTE DIGOXIN POISONING: CASE REPORT AND DETERMINATION OF ELIMINATION HALF-LIFE

Arthur S. Watanabe, Pharm. D.
Instructon or Clinical Pharmacy, University of Utah,
College of Pharmacy. Associate Director, Intermountain Regional Poison Control Center and Drug Information Service

Brent, R. Ekins, B. S., R. Ph.
Clinical Instructor of Clinical Pharmacy, University
of Utah College of Pharmacy. Clinical Pharmacist,
Intermountain Regional Poison Control Center and
Drug Information Service

Joseph C. Veltri, B. S., R. Ph.
Associate Director, Intermountain Regional Poison
Control Center and Drug Information Service

Anthony R. Temple, M. D.
Associate Professor of Pediatrics and Clinical
Toxicology, University of Utah Colleges of Medicine
and Pharmacy. Director, Intermountain Regional
Poison Control Center and Drug Information Service,
Salt Lake City, Utah 84132

ABSTRACT

A 20-month-old, 25 pound, white male child ingested
an unknown quantity of 0.25 mg digoxin tablets.

Serum digoxin levels were measured for 96 hours
following ingestion and the concentrations were plotted
against time. Analysis of the data revealed an elimination half-life of 26 hours, which does not necessarily
confirm a trend reported by others of a shortened half-
life in acute poisoning.

INTRODUCTION

The pharmacokinetics of therapeutic dosages of digoxin have been well studied in adults (2,3), but there
is little information about digoxin kinetics following an acute overdose, especially in the pediatric
patient. In the management of any acute drug overdose
case, it is important to recognize that the expected
pharmacokinetic behavior of a drug may be different
from that seen in the therapeutic situation. This
has been suggested in the literature for digoxin (4-7).
Unfortunately, there are only a limited number of documented cases available to evaluate this situation and
most of these are adult patients. These cases do not
uniformly report the same parameters, treatments performed, or the length of time serum concentrations
were followed. These inconsistencies indicate that
in every case there may not be adequate data to determine an accurate elimination half-life following an
acute overdose. In this paper, we report a case of
acute digoxin intoxication in a 20 month old infant
male, the measurement of serial digoxin levels, and
an estimation of the elimination half-life.

CASE REPORT

A 20 month old, 25 pound, previously healthy white
male was found sitting on the floor with various medications strewn about. A survey of the available
bottles showed the following: multivitamins without
iron, vitamin E, calcium, quinidine, and digoxin
(Lanoxin [R]). The strength of the Lanoxin [R] was
0.25 mg per tablet. Upon finding the boy, the parents
were unable to estimate the amount of missing tablets
for any of the products, and the parents did not think
the child had done anything more than suck on the
tablets. One hour after eating dinner, however, the
child suddenly became nauseated and experienced
spontaneous vomiting. The vomitus contained small
white particles resembling tablet fragments. The

parents then called the Intermountain Regional Poison
Control Center. They were instructed on the use of
ipecac syrup and emesis was induced successfully in
the home, and occurred within 15 minutes, but no additional pill fragments were found. The child was then
referred to the University of Utah Medical Center for
further evaluation and supportive care.

On arrival at the emergency room the child was having dry vomiting, was pale but alert. The physical
examination revealed a pulse rate varying between
60-150 per minute and was irregular. The blood pressure was 100/44. The remainder of the examination
was unremarkable. An initial electrocardiogram showed
first degree atrioventricular block as well as runs of
atrial tachycardia. The child was transferred to the
cardiac care unit where he was administered quarter-
normal saline in five percent dextrose with 40 mEq of
KCl intravenously at a rate of 45 cc/hr. Ten grams of
activated charcoal was given orally and the child was
placed on continuous EKG monitoring. Subsequent EKG
rhythm strips demonstrated varying periods of nodal
tachycardia with rates of up to 150 per minute alternating with 2:1 AV block with a ventricular rate of
60-70 per minute. Additionally, the patient had
periods of normal junctional rhythm with first degree
atrioventricular block with a rate of 100-125 per
minute present. Admitting laboratory data included:
serum sodium 139 mEq/l, serum potassium 5.0 mEq/l,
serum chloride 107 mEq/l, serum carbon dioxide content
19 mEq/l, serum creatinine 0.4 mg/dl, blood urea nitrogen 12 mg/dl, serum glucose 117 mg/dl, serum
calcium 10.0 mg/dl, albumin 4.8 gm/dl, hemoglobin
concentration 12.3 gm/dl, hematocrit 37.9%, white
blood count 9900/mm^3 with normal differential, red
blood count 4.66 million/cu.mm and a serum quinidine
of 1.7 mcg/ml, (therapeutic range 4-8 mcg/ml). The
initial digoxin level drawn 3½ hours after ingestion
was 12.0 ng/ml ($\pm$ .2, normal range 0.8-2.0 ng/ml).
No other drugs were found on analysis. Five hours

after ingestion the patient had a pulse rate between
50 and 60 which responded to atropine sulfate (0.1 mg
I.V.), which was repeated twice thereafter to increase
the heart rate. The AV block persisted for approximately 30 hours. The child developed no other symptoms and was discharged on the third day following
ingestion. At 96 hours following the ingestion, the
child was seen again for a routine check-up and a
final blood sample was drawn.

METHODS

Serum samples were drawn at $3\frac{1}{2}$, 12, 36, 60 and 96
hours postingestion and were assayed for digoxin concentrations by radioimmunoassay as described elsewhere (7), using the Quantitope ^{R} ^{125}I-Digoxin
Radioimmunoassay Kit Method* and all were assayed in
triplicate. All determinations were performed by
the Nuclear Medicine Laboratory of the University of
Utah Medical Center.

Since digoxin appears to follow first order elimination kinetics (1) the following equations were
used to calculate the beta (B) or elimination half-
life. Equation 1-A represents the equation that
defines a first order reaction.

$$C_p = C_po\ e^{-kt} \qquad\qquad \text{1-A}$$

Where C_po is the concentration at time zero, C_p is
the concentration at some time after time zero, e is
the base of the natural logarithm, k is the beta
elimination rate constant, and t is the time after

---

*Quantitope ^{R} ^{125}I-Digoxin Radioimmunoassay Kit is
manufactured by Kallestad Laboratories, Inc., Chaska, MN

time zero. Solving for the half-life $(t_{\frac{1}{2}})$ this equation becomes:

$$t_{\frac{1}{2}} = \cfrac{\ln \cfrac{C_p o}{C_p}}{k} \qquad\qquad \text{1-B}$$

Solving equation 1-B where $\cfrac{C_p o}{C_p} = 2$

the equation becomes:

$$t_{\frac{1}{2}} = \frac{\ln 2}{k} = \frac{.693}{k} \qquad\qquad \text{1-C}$$

RESULTS

The serum concentrations versus time following ingestion are summarized in Table 1, and these values are plotted on semi-logarithmic scale as shown in Figure 1. The slope of the regression line representing the last four values was calculated by the method of least squares and the apparent serum elimination half-life of digoxin was calculated using equation 1-C, where the slope of the regression line represents the derived beta elimination constant. The first value was not used in the determination of elimination half-life since it was assumed to represent the absorption/distribution phase. The half-life for this 20 month old child was calculated to be 26.0 hours.

DISCUSSION

Previous reports in the literature have suggested
that in the acute overdose situation, the elimination
half-life for digoxin is shorter than that expected
for chronic toxicity or normal therapeutic doses (4-7).
The mean half-life values found for normal infants and
children are 32.5 and 38 hours, respectively, and are
not considered significantly different from those found
in adults with normal renal function (2,3). The literature reports a range of half-life values in acute
digoxin poisonings ranging from 6 hours to greater than
35 hours for adults (age range 17-78 years) and one
case of a 2½ year old boy with a reported half-life
value of 12 hours (7). Unfortunately, in many of
these acutely poisoned cases, insufficient data may
have been collected to accurately determine if the reported half-life values reflect only the elimination
half-life or partially the absorption-distribution
phase as well.

Our patient who had ingested an undertermined quantity of digoxin did not necessarily demonstrate a
shortened elimination half-life as expected from the
literature. Although different assay methods were
utilized, our half-life value of twenty six hours
falls within the normal half-life range reported by
Dungan et. al. (range 18-48 hours) (2). We can offer
no definitive explanation for the great variation in
the literature for reported half-lives following an
acute overdose. Inconsistent data gathering and
different assay methods and techniques may have some
influence as well as a normal range of intrapatient
half-life variation. Estimations of serum elimination
half-lives which include absorption-distribution phase
values may contribute to artificially shortened values.
In addition, our patient was given activated charcoal
which has been documented to inhibit the absorption of
therapeutic doses of digoxin (9). The influence of
this variable on assuring that this calculated half-

life represents only the elimination half-
life is not fully known. Shortened half-life values in
the acute overdose situation might also be the result of
prolonged oral absorption or a reduced volume of distribution secondary to tissue binding saturation. Some
drugs may demonstrate concentration dependent half-lives
which may result in different half-life values at different phases of elimination as postulated for digoxin
by one author (7). Another author reports the opposite
effect where the apparent half-life shortened as time
progressed (5). Since half-life values may be of pre-
dictive value in the management of drug overdose,
further study is indicated to clarify the apparent
problem of varying half-life values in the acute digoxin
overdose situation, particularly in pediatric patients.

TABLE I

SERUM DIGOXIN CONCENTRATION vs. TIME POST-INGESTION

12.0 ng/ml	3½ hrs
5.5 ng/ml	12 hrs
3.5 ng/ml	36 hrs
1.9 ng/ml	60 hrs
0.6 ng/ml	96 hrs

REFERENCES

1. Smith TW, Haber E: Digitalis (4 parts). *N Engl J Med* 289:945-951; 289:1010-1015; 289:1003-1072; 289:1125-1129, 1973.

2. Dungan WT, Doherty JE, Harvy C, et al: Tritiated digoxin XVIII-studies in infants and children. *Circ* 46:983, 1972.

3. Hernandez A, Burton RM, Pagtakham RD, et al: Pharmacodynamics of H-digoxin in infants. *Pediatrics* 44:418, 1969.

4. Bertler A, Gustafson A, Redfors A: Massive digoxine intoxication. *ACTA Med Scand* 194:245, 1973.

5. Hobson JD, Zettner A: Digoxin serum half-life following suicidal digoxin poisoning. *JAMA* 223:147, 1973.

6. Rumack BH, Wolfe RR, Gikfrich H: Phenytoin (diphenylhydantoin) treatment of massive digoxine overdose. *Brit Heat J* 36:405, 1974.

7. Smith TW, Willerson JT: Suicidal and accidental digoxin ingestion. *Circ* 44:29, 1971.

8. Smith TW, Butler VP Jr, Haber E: Determination of therapeutic and toxic digoxin concentrations by radioimmunoassay. *N Engl J Med* 281:1212, 1969.

9. Hartel G, Manninen V, Reissek P: Treatment of digoxin intoxication. *Lancet* 2:158, 1973.

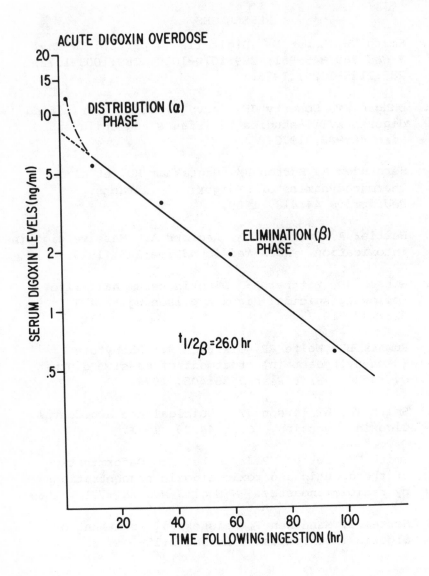

Figure 1. Semilogarithmic plot of serum digoxin
concentrations versus time following
an acute digoxin overdose.

POISON CENTER FUNCTIONS: AN APPROACH TO QUALITY CONTROL

William O. Robertson, M.D.
Director, Poison Control Center
Children's Orthopedic Hospital

ABSTRACT

The recent decade has documented increasing interest in quality assessment in the health field; techniques based on both "input" and "output" measures of the health care process have been espoused. Current interest is focusing on an approach to quality control by professional organizations via certification examinations; such is an input measure.

A contrasting approach utilizing output measures exclusively will be described. Pilot investigations in each of the areas under consideration will be summarized; both outside assessment of the "Center-Consumer" interchange and measures of the consumer's change in behavior will be stressed; poison centers afford unique models permitting quality control assessment of innovations in management as well as modifications of staffing patterns provided by health professionals. A plea will be made that more emphasis be focused on assessment of output in the future--versus exclusive concentration on input measures.

Today, as never before, efforts at quality control are burgeoning throughout Medicine. Most measures continue to be directed toward assessing elements that *produce* medical services--e.g., as is shown in Table 1, the training or qualifications of the individual health care practitioner or his continuing education activities, the physical features or staffing characteristics of the health care institution, the comprehensiveness and

the range of services offered, etc. Such are termed
"effort" or *"input"* criteria. All too few measures are
directed toward assessing elements that *result* from
those medical services (or are assumed to result there-
from)--e.g., immunization rates, age-specific mortality
rates, life expectancies, etc. Such are customarily
termed *"effect"* or *"output"* criteria.

A conventional assumption is that input criteria will
correlate with output criteria. Unfortunately, contradictory data deluge policymakers on this point. For
example, the lowest maternal and infant mortality rates
occur in those states with the lowest ratio of specialists and/or physicians to population, the fewest medical
centers and the least antibiotic usage. Recurrence
rates following inguinal herniorrhaphy do not differ as
a function of the individual surgeon's training and
measurements of interns' learning do not correlate with
either the stature or status of their training insti-
tutions.

Particularly as the Academy of Clinical Toxicology
and American Association of Poison Control Centers are
considering a certification process for Poison Center
personnel, it is timely to pose this question: Might
it not be more effective to accredit Poison Centers by
measuring their corporate outputs than to certify their
individual health practitioners by simply measuring
inputs? Phrased differently, as long as a Center functions effectively and efficiently in accomplishing specified objectives, need we care about the qualifications of those who work there? Let me elaborate on
some outputs or some outcomes we feel are susceptible
to measurement.

In 1975, our Seattle Poison Center--staffed by as
many as 26 different people on any given weekend--
answered more than 25,000 phone calls. For obvious
resaons we have had a continuing concern about the
quality of our performances. While some would propose
only input or effort criteria ought be measured--i.e.,

insist only an R.N. answer the phone--we have chosen instead to look at several effect or output measures, as shown in Table II. First I will describe our techniques--then the results.

Measure #1: Validation of use of information sources.

On each phone contact sheet, space is provided for recording the information source used; while initially completion of this portion of the record was inadequate, recent staff cooperation has permitted assessment of correlations between advice given and information sources used--as well as the appropriateness of the source used.

Measure #2: Caller's compliance with our instructions.

As an example of this approach, a pharmacy graduate completing his third year of medical school was employed to visit the homes of 20 consecutive callers who (1) reported an accidental salicylate ingestion in a child less than 5 years of age, (2) reported having no syrup of ipecac in the home at the time, (3) were requested to purchase syrup of ipecac, and (4) were verified as having provided the Center with an accurate phone number and street address. The student simply visited each home--unannounced--explained his association with the Center, inquired as to the condition of the child, and then asked to examine the syrup of ipecac bottle which hopefully had been secured.

Measure #3: Assessment of staff behavior in telephone conversations.

Tape recording equipment has been purchased and installed. It is activated by incoming phone calls; a fifteen-second-interval beep signals the "bug" is

operative. Thus, actual records of telephone conversations are available for content analysis. Two approaches
toward such analysis are being explored; the first
relates to content; the second to process.

Regarding content, certain standards have been
adopted for use by the staff--e.g., specific detailed
recommendations regarding the use of syrup of ipecac,
the management of hydrocarbon ingestions, plant ingestions, cosmetic ingestions, etc. With the tape
recordings available, it has become a simple task for
the Director of the Center and the Charge Nurse--in-
itially on a routine basis and subsequently on a sampling basis--to compare the content of the phone conversation with the previously enumerated criteria.
(The actual review is carried out during commuting time
to and from work via a portable tape recorder.) Thus,
a staff compliance rate is able to be calculated.

Regarding process, i.e., the manner of the telephone
conversation itself, almost no experimental studies
were able to be uncovered on this subject (despite extensive efforts) that support or attempt to support
one versus another technique of telephone answering.
Consequently, we prepared, after extensive discussion,
a list of five qualitative measures which we felt were
important for "good" phone answering behavior. We then
searched existant tapes to locate conversations which
exhibited both "good" and "bad" telephone behavior. A
series of conversations were dubbed onto yet another
cassette and validation of the appraisal technique undertaken. With the help of groups of parents of young
children--largely but not exclusively mothers--and
subsequently medical and nursing students as well as
graduate nurses--we prepared definitions of the five
qualitative measures, made them available for reading
by "panels" who in turn listened to the conversations
in sequence with a pause between each during which they
graded each performance on a scale of one to five against
the specified characteristics. The purpose was to

assess the consistency and reproduceability of the grade; once the technique was found to be satisfactory, it has been available on an on-going basis to use as a source of constructive criticism for participating staff.

Measure #4:   Response of staff to "contrived" cases.

Begun before installation of the tape equipment and recently expanded in scope, yet another appraisal technique has been undertaken. At first the Director, and subsequently other individuals would call the Center posing as a distraught parent or parent surrogate seeking help or information with reference to a specific issue--potential toxicity, recommended therapy, identification of generic names, etc. While initially the responses were not formally quantified, recently, with the knowledge and cooperation of all ten Centers throughout our state and the assistance of the State Coordinator of Poison Centers, individual calls using the same approach have been placed to each of the centers throughout the state and responses assessed by a battery of four listeners against a peer-prepared listing of expectations.

Measure #5:   Assessment of User Opinions

More recently we have been surveying the health care professionals who are users of our information services via a simple questionnaire. Data sought include the time expended by the Center in answering the phone call and in answering questions, the adequacy and completeness of the answers given and their pertinence to treatment.

In summary, five distinct approaches have been used in assessing Seattle Poison Center's performance in accomplishing its information mission--validation of information source used, compliance by callers, assessment of the telephone behavior, response to contrived cases, and professionals' opinions of the adequacy of the Center's performance.

RESULTS

To date, preliminary results of these approaches have been obtained; initially, some "professional resistance" occurred. It diminished rapidly and the process continues with good cooperation.

As Table III shows, measure #1--analysis of information source validation--confirms less than ideal staff behavior; this suggests three points: (1) a persistence of habits limits staff potential, (2) a reluctance of many staff exists to resort to very technical resources --pharmacology texts, biochemical journals, etc., and (3) occasionally staff hesitate to confirm incomplete statements via a secondary source. To date, however, approximately 90% of the sources used would appear to be satisfactory; additional approaches are being devised to refine the methodology involved.

As is noted in Table IV, measure #2--caller compliance --resulted in the student investigator's eventually contacting all 20 subjects and actually seeing syrup of ipecac bottles in 17 of the 20 homes--none of which reported as having had it prior to the call to the Poison Center.

In Table V, measure #3--the analysis of content of tape recordings--showed that in the initial series of 50 consecutive calls wherein a specific standard had been enumerated for staff compliance, 43 had been followed rather explicitly, four generally followed, and three seemingly igonred. Subsequently, oversights were discussed with the staff and staff supervisor, brief teaching tapes (3-4 minutes) were developed to reinforce the sought-for standards so that subsequent sampling of staff compliance has, over a two-year interval, resulted in a better than 85% satisfactory performance—with virtually no diametrically opposed or contrary staff behavior.

Table VI concerns measure #3—analysis of the process of the call itself. We were pleased to find a remarkable agreement among the individuals on the panels who assessed telephone behaviors. A subsequent comparison between lay reactions and professional reactions has revealed no significant differences. As is noted in the table, the five resultant measures are rather simple concepts which apparently are able to be rather closely assessed by virtually any adult observers. Please note the variation on a scale of 5 between two staff members' performances; Subject B was highly trained but gave consistently poor performances. Despite the detection of some "less than ideal" performances via this method, no satisfactory approach has yet been achieved to bring about altered behavior on the part of the participant—which when checked out on subsequent telephone tapes, revealed a significant change in that behavior. Studies continue on this point. It is difficult to "teach an old dog new tricks" —or even a young dog for that matter.

Table VII focuses on measure #4—the response to "contrived" cases and questions. Quantification of responses to certain features—advising the induction of emesis—has been consistently good. In contrast, response on some controversial issues—the management of hydrocarbon ingestions—has shown a wide disparity between and among the various respondants, as is noted in the table. (But even here, when all 10 Centers throughout the State were queried and no single response was duplicated among any of them, each and every Center concluded its call with the recommendation that if all did not go well with the child, they be recontacted and/or the child brought immediately to the Center for further investigation--an exemplary output!) Additional analysis of this technique is now underway.

And finally, as is indicated in Table VIII, we focus on user opinion. Of those respondants who answer, there has been surprisingly favorable response with satisfactory evidence of performance as is shown in the table. The fact that the user use continues to increase --with some 307 calls from health professionals being received in the month of June 1976 (up from 210 a year ago) tends to support a satisfactory professional image of performance.

DISCUSSION

Reflection of the foregoing output measures would support our contention that it is possible to develop quality control programs which rely on measurements or estimates of performance--as those measurements or estimates compare with previously determined criteria. In this instance, the Poison Control Center serves as an easily accessible model in which to examine the basic issue--input versus output assessment--much as it also serves as a unique model for teaching purposes. The language is specific; criteria can be explicit; large numbers of comparable cases exist. As a result, for example, it is possible to report that--on the basis of still limited numbers--experienced and highly trained staff appear to perform no better in their telephone behavior than do many "nonprofessional personnel." As a matter of fact, in the case of one particularly well trained and highly informed individual staff member, a negative correlation was found.

Why do I feel this overall issue is so important? Four reasons stand out. *First*, several well-motivated groups are actively pursuing the establishment of training or testing criteria to be applied against those who

would function in Poison Centers; no doubt much effort
--people, dollars and time--would go into the development of such testing methods--all without good evidence
of a positive correlation between the resultant, pur-
ported "competence" and the individual's subsequent
behavior. Would it not be more profitable to expend
our limited resources in developing techniques to measure actual performance at the outcome level rather than
simply looking at input. *Second*, a variety of professional groups outside and inside of the Poison field
continue to attempt to mount convincing arguments that
only members of their respective guilds are obviously
qualified to lead or carry out their specific health
care mission. Some would hold the thesis for Poison
Centers that "obviously, only experienced physicians
(or clinical toxicologists) should serve as Directors
of Poison Centers," or "only pharmacists should function in providing drug information," or "only nurses
are prepared to deal with patients over the phone,"
etc. Such hypotheses--while perhaps attractive to the
professional guild--simply don't make sense in the
1970's--and won't be accepted by third party payors
unless they are supported by data. Here again the
Poison Control Center lends itself in a unique fashion
to acceptance or refutation of the espoused positions
by analysis of performances as opposed to measures of
qualifications. And *third*, health care costs continue
to skyrocket; as providers of services, health professionals have long held--and continue to hold--that
health care in the U.S. is excellent--and efficient.
Today, as third party payors--as opposed to individual
patients--pick up the tab (and they pick up nearly 90%
of such costs) they tend to ignore testimonials and
seek supporting data, convinced that costs can and must
be contained! Our choice as professionals is then clear;
collect the data, on performance--or prepare to be ig-
nored. And *fourth*, and finally, the process of collecting data, per se, may serve as a creditable defense
against allegations of professional negligence or mal-
practice in the future, and may uncover techniques to

avoid real negligence. At least we would know--and
could act accordingly. Suffice it to say courts don't
expect miracles but they do seek out documentation of
efforts at quality control by the professionals involved
--i.e., real accountability.

SUMMARY

In summary, our Center, feeling deluged with approximately 100 phone calls per day, continues to be concerned about the quality of its performance; I continue
to be skeptical that the training credentials of the
staff necessarily correlate with good subsequent behavior. Rather than focus on attributes or efforts we
have chosen to look at five avenues of approach to assess the performance or outputs of the Center's activ-
ities--as opposed to committing time and efforts exclusively to assessment of inputs. It is strongly urged
that other Centers try this technique, that our professional associations pursue a comparable approach and
consider accrediting Poison Centers by their outputs
rather than simply certifying participants by their
attributes therein. To me, such makes much sense; it
may save many dollars and it provides maximum discretion
to the local scene to manipulate and optimize its resources as *it* sees fit--encouraging professional ingen-
uity and initiative to evolve.

TABLE I

QUALITY CONTROL
INPUT (EFFORT) MEASURES

1. Professional's degrees
2. Grade point average
3. Years of experience
4. Board certification
5. Budget level
6. Continuing education

TABLE II

QUALITY CONTROL
OUTPUT (EFFECT) MEASURES

1. Information source validation
2. Callers' compliance rate
3. Telephone assessment behavior
4. Response to contrived cases
5. Professional users' opinions

TABLE III

INFORMATION SOURCE VALIDATION

Sample: 100 completed forms

Results: 89 satisfactory source
               8 incomplete source
               3 unsatisfactory source

TABLE IV

CALLER'S COMPLIANCE WITH INSTRUCTIONS

CALLER'S COMPLIANCE WITH INSTRUCTIONS

Sample: 20 home visits re ipecac

Results: 17 homes had ipecac
            3 homes had no ipecac

TABLE V

TELEPHONE BEHAVIOR

CONTENT

Sample: 50 consecutive taped calls

Results: Followed specific standard   43
           General concurrence   4
           Ignored standard   3

TABLE VI

TELEPHONE BEHAVIOR

PROCESS

		Subject	
Source:	30 opinions of 6 calls	A	B
		X Value	
1.	Economy of time	4.3	1.4
2.	Warmth of nurse	3.2	1.9
3.	Assuredness	3.7	1.5
4.	Supportiveness	3.4	1.7
5.	Appropriate language	3.6	2.5

TABLE VII

RESPONSE TO CONTRIVED CASES

Sample: 10 Poison Control Centers
          Re: Hydrocarbon

          Clarify history   6
          Check signs   4
          Induce emesis   4
          Gastric lavage   2
          Nothing   4

TABLE VIII

PROFESSIONAL USERS' OPINIONS

Sample: Consecutive opinionaires   N = 30

Results: Prompt answer <3 rings   29

            Identification adequate   29

            Information quickly   22

            Information 100%   19

            Information 50%   5

            Useful in management   26

SERUM CHLORPROPAMIDE LEVELS FOLLOWING ACCIDENTAL INGESTION

W. H. Pitlick, Ph.D.
Assistant Professor, Department of Pharmaceutics,
School of Pharmacy, University of Pittsburgh,
Pittsburgh, Pennsylvania 15261

D. Kurnit, M.D., Ph.D.
Assistant Resident, Children's Hospital of
Pittsburgh, Pittsburgh, Pennsylvania 15261

A. Kenyon, M.D.
Endocrine Fellow, Children's Hospital of
Pittsburgh, Pittsburgh, Pennsylvania 15261

P. Pirakitikulr, M.S.
Teaching Fellow, Children's Hospital of
Pittsburgh, Pittsburgh, Pennsylvania 15261

ABSTRACT

Accidental ingestion of sulfonylureas has been
reported in children. The reports in the literature
are remarkable from two points of view: there are
few if any, reports of chlorpropamide ingestion
in children, and few toxic blood concentrations of
chlorpropamide have been published. The purpose
of this paper is to present a case study illustrating
the relationship between plasma levels of chlorpropamide, glucose clearance, and clinical outcome in a child following ingestion of chlorpropamide.

Chlorpropamide levels were measured in serum
according to the method of Toolan and Wagner.
Initial levels of chlorpropamide were obtained
approximately 36 hours after ingestion, at which
time the serum concentration was 323 micrograms
per ml. During the next 48 hours, serum levels
declined exponentially with a half-life of

*approximately 35 hours. It was found that there
was a significant correlation (p<.01) between serum
chlorpropamide concentrations and the ratio of
blood glucose divided by glucose infusion rate
(reciprocal glucose clearance). Finally, levels of
serum immunoreactive insulin corresponded closely
with serum chlorpropamide concentrations within
the first 48 hours, but following that period
insulin levels remained elevated for several days.
Serum levels of chlorpropamide are extremely
valuable in assessment of a patient's status and
provide input for further decisions regarding
therapy. Severe hypoglycemia as evidenced by the
markedly increased glucose clearance can be successfully monitored and treated. It appears possible to assess a patient's toxicological status
by monitoring glucose clearance.*

INTRODUCTION

Although drug-induced hypoglycemia has occurred
at all ages, sulfonylureas are rarely reported as
etiologic agents of hypoglycemia in children. There
are numerous reports in the literature concerning
hypoglycemic coma in adults following ingestion of
sulfonylureas. In 1972, Chlorpropamide, the
longest-action agent accounted for 45% of the
published reports (1). In 1970, there was a report
of 56 hypoglycemic comas produced by chlorpropamide
within one year, with 53 patients recovering without sequelae, and three fatalities (2). Accidental
ingestion of sulfonylureas has been reported in
three children, and several suicide attempts have
been reported (1). The reports in the literature
are remarkable from two points of view: there are
few if any, reports of chlorpropamide ingestion in
children, and few toxic blood concentrations of
chlorpropamide have been published (3,4). Although
there are several studies which show correlations

between blood glucose lowering and serum chlorpropamide levels, no such studies have been reported
following accidental ingestions of oral hypoglycemics.
The purpose of this paper is to present a case study
illustrating the relationship between plasma levels
of chlorpropamide, glucose clearance, and clinical
outcome in a child following ingestion of chlorpropamide.

Chlorpropamide levels were measured in serum
according to the method of Toolan and Wagner (5).

CASE REPORT

This was the first admission for this 5 9/12-year-
old female who presented with a chief complaint of
seizures and probable drug ingestion. Less than
twenty-four hours prior to admission, the patient
was noted to be irritable. The evening prior to
admission, she was restless at bedtime but did get
to sleep. The following morning, she was found
sleeping on the floor but responded to her grandmother's request that she return to bed. Shortly
thereafter, the grandmother observed a generalized
grand mal seizure with tonic clonic activity of all
extremities, frothing at the mouth, incontinence
of urine, and lip smacking. The patient was un-
arousable after the seizures but her eyes were open
and her pupils dilated. The grandmother could
evoke no response to painful stimuli. The patient
was taken to a community hospital about sixty
minutes after the seizure and there was described
as lethargic and unable to talk. On evaluation
there, the vital signs were normal. The blood glucose
was 40 and her CBC with differential was normal.
She was given 50 cc. of 50% glucose IV push without
significant change in her clinical picture. Pheno-
barbitol, 90 mg. IM, was administered and the patient
was transferred to Children's Hospital for further
evaluation and definitive care.

The admission physical examination disclosed a well-developed, well-nourished female with periodic breathing. She was obtunded but responsive to painful stimuli. The pulse was 100, respiratory rate 19 with a blood pressure of 115/70 and the weight was 23.9 kilograms. Neurologically the child did respond to light touch, pin prick and deep pain; she was not conversive. Her cranial nerves were intact without evidence of palsy; motor function was grossly intact.

The presumptive diagnosis at the time of admission was hypoglycemia secondary to Diabinese ingestion. This impression was confirmed by spectroscopic analysis. Achieving normal glycemia was difficult in this patient. The patient was started on glucagon, 2 mg. per hour IV drip and IV Solu-Cortef, 5 mg. per kg. every six hours. The patient was able to maintain relative normal glycemia by 72-96 hours after admission. She was also started on Phenobarbital 12 mg. per kg. and Dilantin 10 mg. per kg. in an effort to abort the seizures [presumably secondary to hypoglycemia]. In addition she required rectal paraldehyde. An EEG disclosed diffuse slowing consistent with metabolic encephalopathy. A repeat study eleven days after hospitalization and approximately one week after the last seizure was noted was also felt to be abnormal.

DISCUSSION

It is apparent from a plot of serum chlorpropamide concentrations versus time (Fig. 1) that a very large amount of drug on a per kilogram basis had been ingested, though an exact amount could not be ascertained from the patients history. Initial levels of chlorpropamide were obtained approximately 36 hours after ingestion, at which time the serum concentration was 323 micrograms per ml. This delayed hypoglycemic effect has previously been reported in a nondiabetic patient following a suicide attempt with chlorpropamide (4). During the next 48 hours, serum levels declined exponentially with a half-live of approximately 35 hours. This value corresponds favorably with values reported in the literature (3). The remainder of the serum concentration time curve was not suitable for more than elementary pharmacokinetic analysis.

As shown in Fig. 2, it was found that there was a significant correlation ($p < .01$) between serum chlorpropamide concentrations and the ratio of blood glucose divided by glucose infusion rate (reciprocal glucose clearance). The relationship between these two variables was not markedly affected by concomitant administration of glucagon within the 24 to 48 hour period.

Finally, levels of serum immunoreactive insulin corresponded closely with serum chlorpropamide concentrations within the first 48 hours, but following that period insulin levels remained elevated for several days while serum concentrations of chlorpropamide decreased to zero. This is in contrast with the relatively low values of insulin reported in diabetic patients with chlorpropamide induced hypoglycemia (7).

This case illustrates several important points in the diagnosis and management of drug-induced hypoglycemia. First of all, the hypoglycemic effect may be quite prolonged, and peak effects may not be seen until many hours following an ingestion. Serum levels of chlorpropamide are extremely valuable in assessment of a patients status and provide input for further decisions regarding therapy. Severe hypoglycemia as evidenced by the markedly increased glucose clearance can be successfully monitored and treated. In the absence of capabilities for rapid determination of serum concentrations of chlorpropa-

mide, it appears possible to assess a patient's
toxicological status by monitoring glucose clearance.

REFERENCES

1. Stelzer HS: Drug-induced hypoglycemia. *Diabetes*
   21:955, 1972.

2. Agarwal RC, et al: Chlorpropamide-induced hypoglycemia. *Diabetes* 19:376, 1970.

3. Kumar DM, et al: Serum chlorpropamide in drug-
   induced hypoglycemia. *J Assoc Phys India* 21:275,
   1973.

4. Forest JAH: Chlorpropamide overdosage: Delayed
   and prolonged hypoglycemia. *Clin Toxicol* 7:19,
   1974.

5. Toolan TJ, Wagner RL: The physical properties
   of chlorpropamide and its determination in human
   serum. *Ann NY Acad Sci* 74:449, 1959.

6. Dowell RC, Imrie AH: Chlorpropamide poisoning in
   nondiabetics. *Scot Med J* 17:305, 1972.

7. Kumar DM, et al: Insulin and growth hormone in
   chlorpropamide induced hypoglycemia. *Diabetes*
   20:365, 1971.

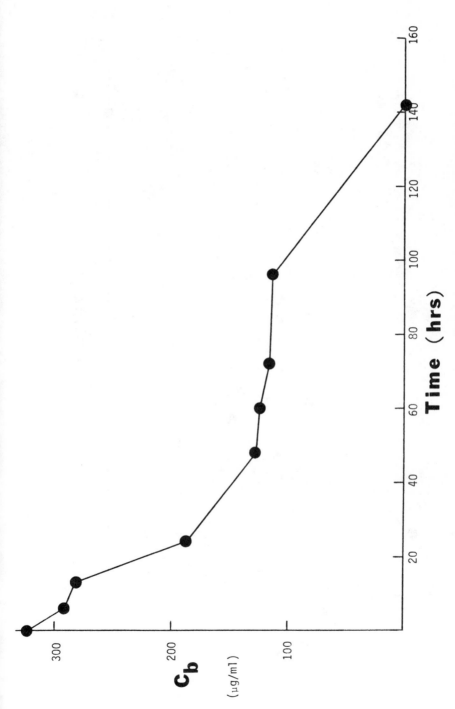

Figure 1. Plot of serum chlorpropamide concentrations in micrograms per ml. versus time. T 1/2 during first 48 hours = 35 hours.

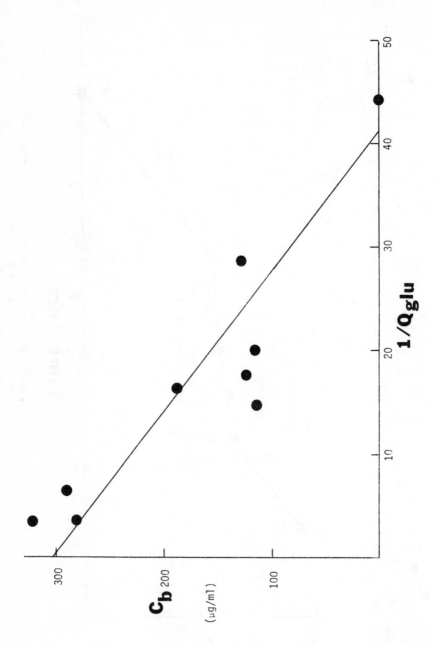

Figure 2. Plot of serum chlorpropamide concentrations (C_b) versus reciprocal glucose clearance (1/Qglu) (Correlation coefficient = 0.913, p<.01).

DIGOXIN - LITHIUM DRUG INTERACTION

W.D. Winters, M.D., Ph.D.
Director, Poison Control Center, Emergency Medicine,
Sacramento Medical Center
Professor of Pharmacology, School of Medicine,
University of California at Davis

David D. Ralph, M.D.
Assistant Professor of Internal Medicine, University
of California at Davis
Associate Director, Poison Control Center, University
of California at Davis

ABSTRACT

Lithium salts and digitalis glycosides are classes
of drugs that share as common properties a narrow toxic/
therapeutic ratio and a propensity to induce cardiac
arrhythmias, even at "therapeutic" blood levels. We
describe a patient taking commonly-used dosages of lith-
ium carbonate and digoxin who presented with increasing
tremulousness, marked confusion, and a severe nodal brad-
ycardia alternating with slow atrial fibrillation. The
lithium blood level was in the toxic range at 2.0 meq/l
and the digoxin level was in the lower therapeutic
range at 0.7 ng/ml at the time of admission when the
patient had a junctional bradycardia at a rate of 52
beats/minute. However, despite discontinuation of both
medicines, the rate fell to 30 the following day, re-
quiring placement of a temporary pacemaker which had to
be kept in place for six days before the patient revert-
ed to normal sinus rhythm. Although the serum potassium
level was always normal, we postulate that the intra-
cellular potassium depletion known to be caused by lith-
ium potentiated the effect of the digoxin and thus led
to a synergistic toxic effect resulting in the prolonged
arrhythmia. This is the first report describing such
a clinical presentation. As lithium salts become more

commonly used in the elderly population, which also has
frequent use of digoxin, increasing numbers of patients
will be at risk for similar arrhythmias.

INTRODUCTION

Three recent case reports describe patients taking
lithium salts for the treatment of psychiatric disorders who developed cardiac arrhythmias consisting of
abnormal sinus node impulse formation (1,2,3). It has
been known for several years that a high percentage of
patients treated with lithium will have reversible changes
in the T waves of their electrocardiograms. Indeed,
Demers (4) showed that all of the patients he carefully
studied with multiple EKG's demonstrated T wave depression. Such an effect was felt to be of little clinical
significance but the description of cardiac arrythmias
due to lithium indicates that its cardiac toxicity may
be of major importance on occasion.

We describe a patient who had prolonged bradyarrhythmias while taking both lithium and digoxin. At the
time of first appearance of the abnormal rhythm his
blood level of lithium was in the toxic range while
his blood level of digoxin was in the usual therapeutic
range. Treatment with lithium may increase the propensity to digitalis-induced arrhythmias by causing
depletion of intracellular potassium. Thus the combination of two agents which may independently pre-
dispose to arrhythmias and which may in addition
potentiate each other creates a situation where serious disorders or cardiac conduction can occur.

CASE REPORT

A 67-year-old Caucasian man was admitted to the hospital on 21 January 1976 because of tremor and increasing disorientation that had developed after he was
placed on lithium carbonate in a nursing home. History

revealed that the patient had been on digoxin 0.125 mg per day for several years because of a previous episode of congestive heart failure felt to be secondary to longstanding hypertension. There was no evidence of previous myocardial infarction. He also had mild chronic obstructive pulmonary disease and chronic lower extremity edema attributed to local venous insufficiency. For several years he had experienced recurrent episodes of depression with one or two occurrences of hypomania. A previous EKG in December 1972 when he was on digoxin alone was normal (Figure 1).

Twelve days before admission because of increasingly withdrawn behavior he was started on 300 mg t.i.d. of lithium carbonate. Four days later the nursing home notes revealed that he had had an excellent response and was "a new man" with increasingly appropriate social interactions. However by four days before admission he began to develop a coarse tremor and over the next two days had steadily increasing confusion, disorientation and worsening of the tremor. A lithium level two days before admission was 2.1 meq/l with a repeat level of 2.0 meq/l the day before admission at which time the vital signs first showed a regular bradycardia at a rate of 52. He was not on diuretics or sodium restriction.

Admission physical revealed an elderly man with a blood pressure of 140/90, pulse 55 and regular, who was confused, uncommunicative and occasionally agitated. Examination further showed a normal thyroid gland, mild gynecomastia, distention of the neck veins, no cardiac gallops, distant breath sounds, and +2 pitting edema of the ankles. There was a coarse resting tremor; reflexes were hyperactive. Hematocrit was 30%, white count 9,900, sodium 131 meq/l, potassium 4.3 meq/l, chloride 106 meq/l, bicarbonate 25 meq/l, BUN 27, creatinine 1.9, and creatinine clearance 38cc/min. T_3 and T_4 were normal. Calcium of 8.2 mg% was normal for the albumin of 3.3. The admission lithium blood level was 2.0 meq/l with a digoxin level of 1.0 ng/ml. Serum magnesium was not measured. Chest X-ray showed mild congestive failure. The first EKG revealed either a slow junctional rhythm or a regularized slow atrial fibrillation at a rate of 50 (Figure 2). No P waves were demonstrable. QRS duration was prolonged at 0.11 seconds; QT interval was normal at 0.40 seconds. There was mild ST depression in leads II, III, aVF, V_5 and V_6 with low voltage. This represented a marked change from the previously normal EKG.

After hospitalization the lithium and digoxin were discontinued and diuresis first with mannitol and subsequently with aminophylline was instituted. Supplemental potassium was given daily and the serium potassium always remained normal. On the second hospital day the lithium level had decreased to 1.8 meq/l and the digoxin level to 0.7 ng/ml but the heart had dropped to a junctional rate of only 30 to 40 responsive only transiently to atropine or isoproterenol infusion. Accordingly a temporary demand cardiac pacemaker was inserted. Over the next five days the lithium and digoxin levels fell at the rate expected for the patient's level of renal function (Table 1). During this time a slow intrinsic rate and conduction delay continued with a gradual increase in the rate (Figures 2, 3, and 4). By the sixth day the patient was in atrial fibrillation with a ventricular response rate of 70 with disappearance of the conduction delay (Figure 5). The lithium level was now 0.4 meq/l with no digoxin detected. The following day the rhythm reverted to normal sinus rhythm with a borderline prolonged PR interval of 0.20 seconds. The pacemaker was then removed. The final EKG on the eighth hospital day showed the PR reduced to 0.18 seconds but ST-T abnormalities persisted (Figure 6).

DISCUSSION

Lithium is a cation which demonstrates a low toxic to therapeutic ratio. Thus blood levels must be monitored closely during therapy to keep the level below 1.5 meq/l. The ratio of intracellular to extracellular lithium is

usually about 0.30 to 0.55 in red blood cells which may
reflect the ratio in nerve cells (5). This ratio may
vary greatly, perhaps being lower in states of active
mania or depression. Accordingly following red cell
rather than blood lithium levels has been proposed as
a better prediction of toxicity. Clinical toxicity is
usually manifest by neuromuscular irritability with trem-
or, hyperreflexia, and by marked CNS abnormalities with
slurred speech, somnolence, occasional agitation, and
progression to coma (6). All of these symptoms are
fully reversible with withdrawal of the drug, but because lithium is extruded from the intracellular space
at a rate only one-tenth that of sodium, the resolution
of clinical toxicity lags behind the fall in blood levels which should average a 50% reduction every one or
two days in patients with normal renal function (7).
Since 95% of lithium is excreted unchanged in the urine
a decrease in renal function will prolong toxicity, a
factor which was probably operative in this patient.

Effects of lithium on the myocardium and electrical
conduction system of the heart are incompletely understood. Several authors have commented that the T wave
flattening in the EKG's of patients on lithium mimics
the classic EKG of potassium depletion (4,8). Extracellular potassium levels are normal in patients on
lithium, but since 97% of the total body potassium is
intracellular, the serum potassium does not reflect
the intracellular concentration. Although various studies sometimes disagree, it is generally held that lithium displaces both sodium and potassium from cells (9).
One patient with lithium intoxication from the use of a
commercial lithium salt substitute who was described
by Hanlon in 1949 had an intraventricular conduction
delay when his serum lithium level was 4.8 meq/l (10).
Singer (9) notes that lithium decreases spontaneous
phase four depolarization of the action potential, in-
duces decremental conduction, and importantly slows conduction through the atrioventricular node and ventricle.
However, the exact effects of chronic lithium adminis-

tration on the human cardiac conduction tissue remain
to be fully described.

Three patients have been reported to have significant
sinus node abnormalities while on lithium (1,2,3).
Eliasen and Anderson (1) reported a patient with second
degree heart block (no blood lithium level reported) who
experienced nodal tachycardia and premature ventricular
contractions with atropine or exercise. Wellens' patient
(2) had a slow irregular sinus rhythm at a rate of 45 per
minute when her lithium level was 1.0 meq/l. His bundle
studies showed a prolongation of the effective refractory period of the right atrium but no change in the conduction through the AV node or in the A-H or H-V intervals or in the width of the QRS. Wilson (3) described
another patient who also developed an irregular sinus
bradycardia. When the blood lithium level was 1.5 meq/l a
His bundle study showed an abnormally slow sinus recovery time. As in the other two patients, all the abnormalities resolved when lithium was discontinued.

Digoxin, of course, is also known to have a narrow
toxic to therapeutic ratio. Toxic atrial and ventricular arrhythmias occur in a large percentage of patients
on digitalis products. Monitoring of serum digoxin levels may decrease the frequency of such arrhythmias (11).
Like lithium, digoxin is also cleared mainly through renal excretion with about 37% daily disappearance with
normal renal function versus about 15% in anuric patients.
Even at therapeutic levels digoxin is associated with a
faster rise of phase four of the transmembrane action
potential and thus increased automaticity and more frequent arrhythmias (12). A slower rise of phase 0, slower
conduction velocity and increased refractory period of
the conduction tissue and especially the AV node can
lead to heart block with escape or re-entrant arrhythmias. Hypokalemia promotes the toxic effects of digoxin (11). Digoxin overdosage may poison the sodium-
potassium pump leading to intracellular potassium depletion.

The patient described in this report had a prolonged episode of a slow junctional rhythm. His arrhythmia may have been due to either simple additive or to additional synergistic actions of lithium and digoxin. The most obvious mechanism of interaction would be that the intracellular potassium depletion caused by lithium enhances digoxin-toxic arrhythmias just as potassium depletion from diuretics would. This is an attractive hypothesis since the EKG of patients on lithium mimics potassium depletion. There are, however, many other possible mechanisms of interaction. For instance, lithium is known to increase serum magnesium levels (13), possibly through extruding magnesium from cells in a manner similar to its effects on potassium. Chronic magnesium depletion has been associated with increased frequency of digitalis-induced arrhythmias (11), and intracellular magnesium depletion from lithium may act similarly. Alternatively, lithium has been said to decrease carbohydrate metabolism in the myocardium with secondarily depressed conduction in the heart (14). Lithium and digoxin may further interact by their effects on the autonomic innervation of the heart or by their actions in depressing the sodium-potassium membrane pump of cardiac cells by interference with the adenyl cyclase which is necessary to the pump (6). The exact nature of the interaction between digoxin and lithium at the cellular level awaits further research.

SUMMARY

In summary, we describe a patient taking lithium and digoxin who had an extended serious arrhythmia. Whatever the mechanism of the interaction between digoxin and lithium on the heart, it is important to be aware that patients on this drug combination are at risk for the development of severe bradyarrhythmias and dangerous escape rhythms. As the popularity of and indications for lithium therapy expand, especially in the older age group, more patients may be exposed to the potential cardiac toxicity of this drug combination.

TABLE I

HOSPITAL COURSE

Hospital Day	Digoxin ng/ml	Lithium meq/l	EKG	CNS Status
-1	--	2.1	--	tremor, confusion
1	1.0	2.0	JB 52, IVCD low voltage abnormal ST-T	hyperreflexia
2	0.7	1.8	JB 37	somnolent
3	--	1.3	JB 50	--
4	--	0.8	JB 50	less confused
6	less than 0.5	0.4	AFib 70 IVCD	tremor and hyper-reflexia have resolved
7	--	--	NSR, PR 0.20	--
8	--	0.2	NSR, PR 0.18 abnormal ST-T	oriented

JB - junctional bradycardia

IVCD - intraventricular conduction delay

AFib - atrial fibrillation

NSR - normal sinus rhythm

REFERENCES

1. Eliasen P, Anderson M: Sinoatrial block during lithium treatment. *European J Cardiol* 3:2:97, 1975.

2. Wellens HJ, Cats VM, Duren DR: Symptomatic sinus node abnormalities following lithium carbonate therapy. *Am J Med* 59:285, 1975.

3. Wilson JR, Kruas ES, Bailas MM, et al: Reversible sinus-node abnormalities due to lithium carbonate therapy. *N Engl J Med* 294:1223, 1976.

4. Demers RG, Heninger GR: Electrocardiographic T-wave changes during lithium carbonate treatment. *JAMA* 218:381, 1971.

5. Mendels J, Frazer A: Alterations in cell membrane activity in depression. *Am J Psychiatry* 131:11, 1974.

6. Baldessarini RJ, Lipinski JF: Lithium salts: 1970-1975. *Ann Int Med* 83:527, 1975.

7. Thomsen K, Schou M: Renal lithium excretion in man. *Am J Physiol* 215:823, 1968.

8. Kochar MH, Wang RI, D'Cunha GF: *J Electrocard* 4:371, 1971.

9. Singer I, Rotenberg D: Mechanisms of lithium action. *N Engl J Med* 289:254, 1973.

10. Hanlon LW, Romaine M, Gilroy FJ, et al: *JAMA* 139:688, 1949.

11. Smith TW, Haber E: Digitalis. *N Engl J Med* 289:945, 1973.

13. Birch NJ: The effects of lithium on plasma magnesium. *Brit J Psychiat* 116:461, 1970.

14. Riciutti MA, Lisi KR, Damato AN: A metabolic basis for the electrophysiological effects of lithium. *Circulation* 44:217, 1971.

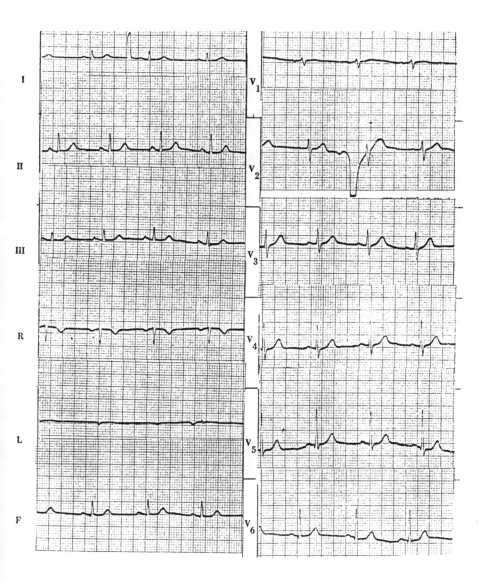

Figure 1. EKG of 12/72 When Patient Was on Digoxin

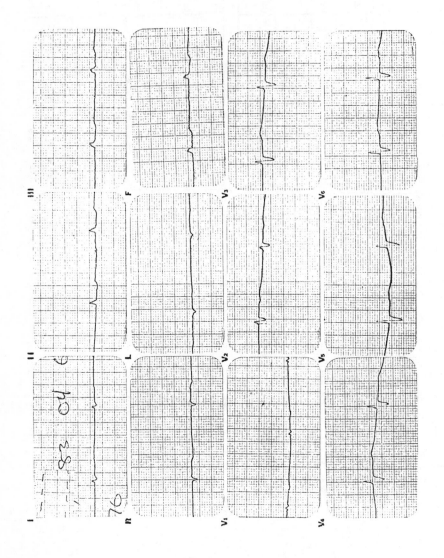

Figure 2. EKG on Admission

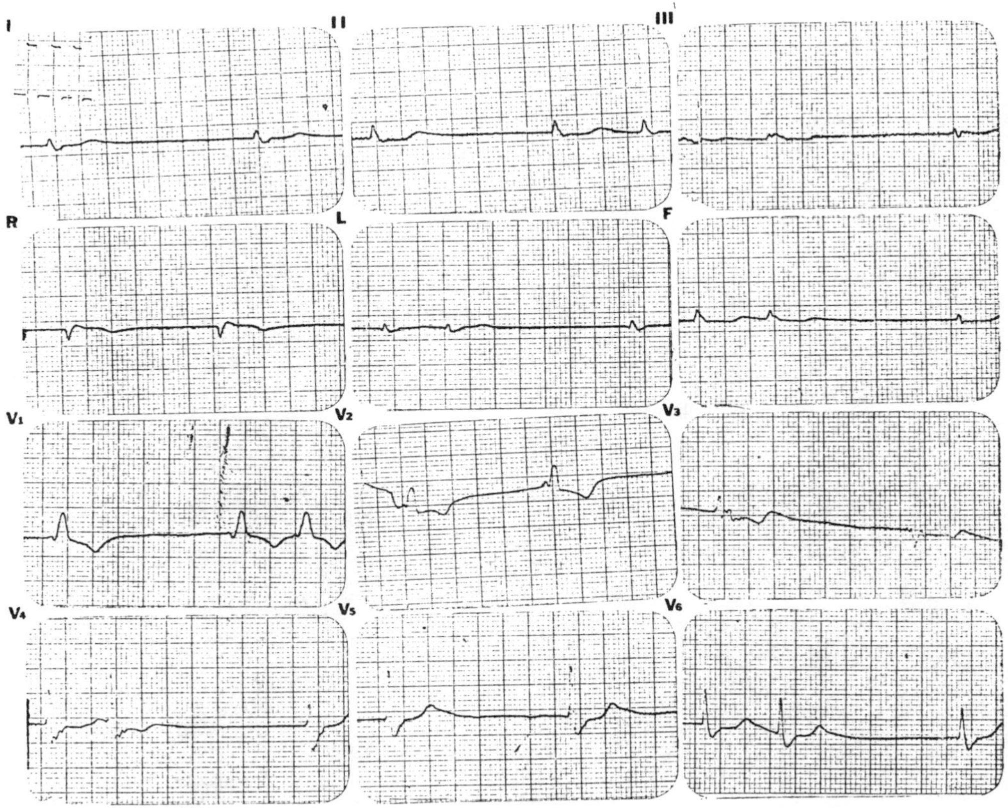

Figure 3. EKG: Day 2

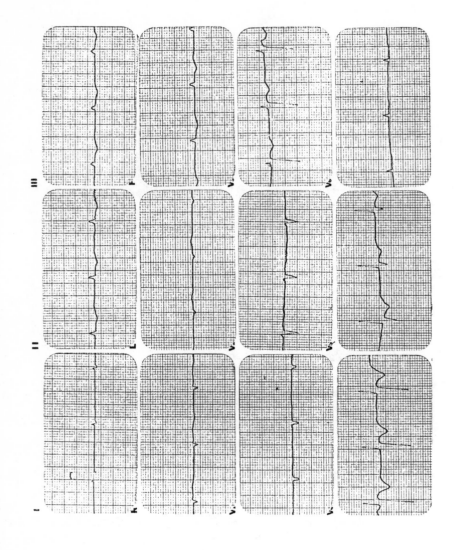

Figure 4. EKG: Day 3

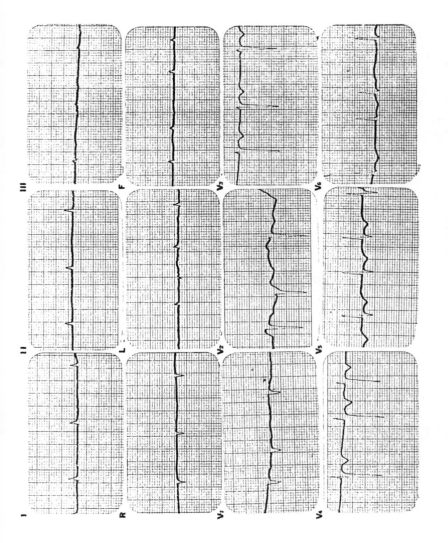

Figure 5. EKG: Day 6

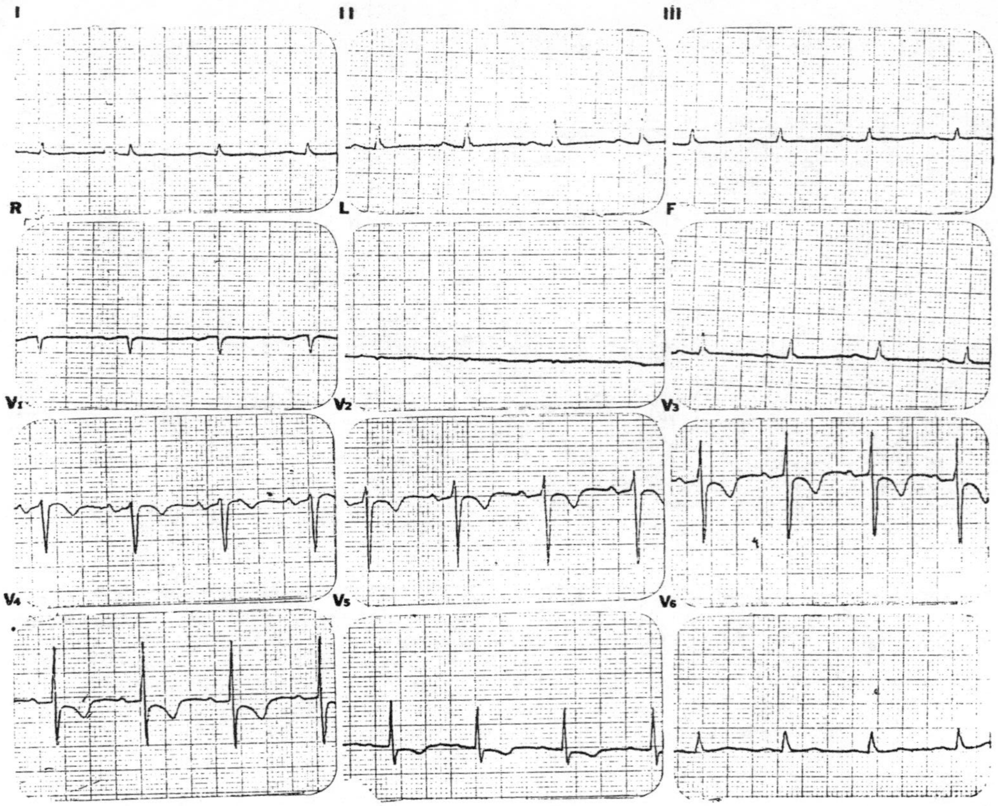

Figure 6. EKG: Day 8

STATUS EPILEPTICUS OR REPETITIVE SEIZURES FOLLOWING TOXIC INGESTION

Gary S. Wasserman, D.O.
Pediatrician in Ambulatory Medicine and Clinical
Toxicologist, The Children's Mercy Hospital, Kansas City
Instructor of Pediatrics, University of Missouri School
of Medicine at Kansas City

Vernon A. Green, Ph.D.
Chief of Toxicological Services at The Children's Mercy
Hospital, Kansas City
Professor, School of Medicine, University of Missouri
at Kansas City

R. Eugene Baska, M.D.
Neurologist-in-Chief, Children's Mercy Hospital,
Kansas City
Associate Professor of Neurology and Pediatrics,
University of Missouri School of Medicine

ABSTRACT

Three children had status epilepticus or repetitive
seizures for approximately two hours before proper
treatment was initiated. Two of these children were
intoxicated with the tricyclic imipramine HCl (Tofranil)
and the other with the thioxanthene chlorprothixene
(Taractan). All had complete recovery, to what their
parents considered normal behavior, within 24-72 hours.
This excellent prognosis has not previously been appreciated in the literature. A MEDLINE search of the
recent English literature reveals no singular article
discussing status epilepticus or repetitive seizures
as a consequence of a toxic ingestion. A list of the
common possible convulsion-producing agents will be
presented. Brief case reviews will be discussed.

'Status epilepticus' may be defined in various ways. It may be classically defined as a seizure lasting longer than thirty minutes or repetitive seizures without an intervening period of consciousness. Convulsive (motor) status may result in death or permanent neurologic impairment. Nonconvulsive status (nonmotor, or so called petit mal status) though important, does not present the same pressing and immediate problems. Recently the term prolonged seizure activity has been used to express continuous generalized or focal seizures lasting ten minutes or longer, as well as three or more separate seizures within the prior half-hour (1).

Convulsive status epilepticus is a medical emergency, requiring not only prompt therapy but also simultaneous investigation of etiology, for in most published series the prognosis is far more grave in the symptomatic group when known epileptics are excluded (2,3,4).

Vascular, traumatic, and metabolic causes are frequent and brain tumor has been stressed as a common cause of unheralded status (the syndrome of isolated status epilepticus) in a previously healthy patient (5). Also, drug withdrawal, infections of the central nervous system (CNS) and encephalopathies such as Reye's syndrome must be added to the list of frequent etiologies.

Drugs and chemicals may induce convulsion by various mechanisms which include a direct effect on CNS, a response to the stimulation of peripheral receptors (e.g. carotid sinus), or by oxygen deprivation (hypoxia or anoxia). Convulsions are dangerous because the patient may die of anoxia or respiratory failure or he may sustain permanent brain damage.

The immediate treatment is basically the same for seizures of any etiology, however, seizures secondary to toxic ingestion often do not respond to the usual anticonvulsant treatment regimen. With advances, in recent years, in the use of antidotal therapy in clinical toxicology, many of these seizure cases can be aborted within minutes or even seconds if the exact etiology is known and the proper antidote administered. Convulsions are usually followed by coma and respiratory depression and the physician should be cautious about the use of antidotes which may further depress the CNS.

It is not within the scope of this paper to discuss treatment of convulsions and the reader is referred to articles on the subject (6,7).

In young children unheralded status appears to be more common than in adults, as does fatality from the seizures themselves (5 to 10%). Permanent neurologic impairment is frequent (37%), as in ensuing epilepsy (57%)(8). Reports involving large numbers of patient cases and especially pediatric series are rare.

In our children's hospital over 60,000 patients visit the emergency room annually. In 1975, three patients were seen with unheralded status epilepticus secondary to accidental drug ingestion. This represents 25% of the cases of status epilepticus (43% of unheralded status). These three cases actually presented within a six month period.

In the recent literature, as well as in most standard textbooks of toxicology, pediatrics, neurology, child neurology, and epilepsy there is scant mention of intoxication as a cause of status. A thorough review of the English literature and partial world literature (MEDLINE, Cumulated Index Medicus 1966-1976, and Excerpta Medica, Epilepsy Abstracts 1945-1976) reveals that there is no singular article discussing the importance of toxic ingestion as a cause of prolonged seizure activity.

Case Summary No. 1

After this six-year-old girl, weighing 24 kilograms, became semicomatose and had a grand mal seizure, it was discovered that an hour earlier she ingested imipramine (29 Tofranil tablets, 725 mg) that she and her sib took from mother's purse.

She was given 90 mg of phenobarbital I.M. at the referring hospital. She seizured during the ambulance ride and was seizuring on admission to the Emergency Room at Children's Mercy Hospital. Five milligrams of Valium I.V. did not stop the seizure but 0.5 mg of physostigmine salicylate (Antilirium) I.V. was effective. No major motor seizure activity recurred. Physostigmine was given as needed, but no further anticonvulsant treatment was used.

This patient had CNS depression, repetitive seizures, cardiac arrhythmia, and hypotension. She became coherent at approximately 14 hours post ingestion, but did not totally recover until 48 hours post ingestion.

Case Summary No. 2

This two and one-half-year-old girl, weighing 13 kilograms, ingested imipramine (25 Tofranil tablets, 625 mg) from a container that was not securely closed. One hour later she had a grand mal seizure and was treated with Valium (5 mg) I.V. at the referring hospital. During her ride by family car to Children's Mercy Hospital she developed status epilepticus for 20 minutes which was stopped in our emergency room with 0.5 mg physostigmine salicylate (Antilirium) I.V. She suffered no further seizures. Her lavage fluid drug screen was strongly diagnostic-positive for imipramine. Physostigmine was used as needed, but no other anticonvulsant regimen was necessary.

This patient had CNS depression, unheralded status

epilepticus, cardiac arrhythmia, and aspiration pneumonitis as well as other complications. She began to respond to external stimuli approximately 10 hours post ingestion, but needed a few days to totally recover.

Case Summary No. 3

Unknown to her family this 21-month-old girl, weighing 10 kilograms, ingested chlorprothixene (Taractan tablets, 50 mg, amount unknown). A few hours later she developed repetitive seizures and was transferred to Children's Mercy Hospital with no treatment initiated by the referring hospital.

She suffered status epilepticus for the next hour. During part of this time in the emergency room she was treated with a total of 27 mg of Valium I.V.; 100 mg phenobarbital I.V.; and 200 mg Dilantin I.V.; in addition to dextrose, calcium, and bicarbonate for seizures of unknown etiology. A urine drug screen was diagnostic. She was maintained on Dilantin and phenobarbital, and no further seizure activity was noted. She was discharged on phenobarbital therapy which was tapered and later discontinued.

This patient had coma, unheralded status epilepticus, and aspiration pneumonitis. She began to respond to external stimuli approximately 11 hours post ingestion, but did not totally recover for a few days.

It should be understood that our immediate treatment included a thorough gastric lavage, charcoal, and the use of a saline cathartic.

One year followup (complete child development evaluation) on all three cases revealed normal development with no evidence of any sequelae. This excellent prognosis for status epilepticus secondary to toxic ingestion has not previously been mentioned in the literature.

Numerous agents may induce convulsive activity, but fortunately the seizures produced by the toxic doses of most of these drugs and chemicals do not mimic status. The following is a list of agents which are more likely to cause prolonged seizure activity.

Stimulants:
   Amphetamines - methamphetamine, etc.
   Camphor - gum, spirits
   Tricyclic antidepressants -imipramine, amitriptyline
   Iproniazid and related compounds - Marsilid, Parnate
                                    MAO inhibitor)

Depressants:
   Phenothiazines - Thorazine, promazine
   Haloperidol - Haldol
   Chlorprothixene - Taractan
   Phencyclidine - Sernyl (PCP)

Narcotics:
   Methyl morphine - codeine
   Proproxyphene HCl - Darvon
   Narcotic abstinence syndrome

Miscellaneous agents:
   Isoniazid hydrazine
   Phenol
   Salicylates
   Halogenated hydrocarbon pesticides - chlordane
   Quaternary ammonium compounds - benzalkonium
                                  chloride
   Boric acid and related compounds
   Ergot derivatives
   Drug withdrawal - barbiturate, phenytoin, ethyl
                    alcohol

In summary, the physician should be alert to the possibility of toxic ingestion in the previously healthy patient who presents with status epilepticus, especially in children. Identification of the intoxi-

cant may well lead to specific antidotal therapy.
These cases may have a far better prognosis than the
literature suggests for unheralded status.

REFERENCES

1. Prensky AL, Raff MC, More MJ, et al: Intravenous diazepam in the treatment of prolonged seizure
activity. *New Eng J Med* 276:779, 1967.

2. Celesia GG: Modern concepts of status epilepticus. *JAMA* 235:1571-1574, 1976.

3. Janz D: Conditions and causes of status epilepticus. *Epilepsia* 2:170-177, 1961.

4. Oxbury JM, Whitty CWM: Causes and consequences
of status epilepticus in adults. *Brain* 94:733-744,
1971.

5. Oxbury JM, Whitty CWM: The syndrome of isolated
epileptic status. *J Neurol Neurosurg Psychiat*
34:182-184, 1971.

6. Greene CA, Rao VS: Current concepts-Status epilepticus. *Nebr S Med J* pp 663-666, November 1970.

7. Conomy JP, McNamara JO: Emergency management
of the patient with seizures, Part I: Generalized
status epilepticus. *Postgrad Med* 55:2, 71-74, 1974.

8. Aircardie J, Chevrie JJ: Convulsive status epilepticus in infants and children: A study of 239
cases. *Epilepsia* 11:187-197, 1970.

A FAST-ACTING ORAL LIQUID EMETIC AGENT

James E. Weaver, Ph.D.
The Proctor & Gamble Company, Sharon Woods Technical
Center, Cincinnati, Ohio 45241

ABSTRACT

Routine emetic studies on dogs performed during the
toxicologic evaluation of built detergent formulations
have shown these products to be prompt-acting, potent
emetic agents. A study of ingredients of detergent
preparations indicated the phosphate builders primarily
were responsible for the emetic activity. In contrast,
Syrup of Ipecac, U.S.P.--the emetic agent of choice for
household and emergency room use--is a slow-acting,
rather unreliable drug.

FORMULATION

Based upon preliminary experiments, it was determined
that a concentration of approximately 20% phosphate
would be required if a reliable emetic effect was to
be obtained at a reasonable dose volume. The relatively
low water solubility of sodium tripolyphosphate (STP),
the most widely-used phosphate builder, precluded its
use as the sole active; therefore, a combination of STP
and a second popular detergent builder was tested and
found to be effective. The combination of 12% STP and
8% tetrapotassium pyrophosphate (TKPP) is the active
system for the Liquid Emetic Agent formula.

The 20% phosphate solution has a bitter, salty taste.
Therefore, elementary attempts to develop a palatable
formulation were made. A flavoring agent was selected
by human adult volunteers who tasted completed formulas
and ranked their flavors according to overall taste.
Of five flavoring systems tested, imitation strawberry,

in combination with saccharin sweetener, best masked the taste of the phosphate solution. Investigations proceeded using the strawberry-flavored material. This formula is shown in Table I.

EMETIC ACTIVITY

Emetic activity was studied using purebred beagle dogs of approximately 7 to 15 months of age (Table II). Test materials were administered undiluted by intra-gastric intubation. Unless otherwise stated, animals were fasted for approximately 16 hours and deprived of water for two hours prior to dosing.

These tests utilized a Latin Square design. Groups of one male and one female dog were given LEA, a dis-tilled water control, or LEA preceded by subcutaneous doses of 2 mg/kg chlorpromazine hydrochloride solution (CPZ) one-half hour before the administration of the emetic agent. Syrup of Ipecac was tested in similar fashion for reference. The doses of LEA and Syrup of Ipecac employed produced emesis in about 80-90% of the animals dosed. CPZ was given to explore the mechanism of emesis introduction. CPZ effectively blocks the chemoreceptor trigger zone in the medulla, as indicated by the prevention of emesis from intravenous apomorphine; therefore, if the emetic agent induced emesis by a cen-tral action in the chemoreceptor trigger zone, pretreat-ment with CPZ would block the emetic response.

The effects of LEA, in doses of 0.15 ml/kg (30 mg/kg based upon total phosphate), were unaffected by pre-treatment with CPZ. Emesis, when produced, occurred promptly. In comparison, (Table III) emetic effects of Syrup of Ipecac (0.35 ml/kg), manifested themselves much more slowly, lasted for a considerably longer pe-riod of time, and were significantly antagonized by pretreatment with CPZ ($p < 0.01$).

Based upon the above, it was estimated that a total of LEA of 5 ml, given to dogs of approximately 10 kg weight, would prove effective as well as safe. As shown in Table IV, total doses of 5 ml of LEA were given to groups of nonfasted dogs or of nonfasted dogs which had been pretreated with intragastric administration of 240 ml of milk one-half hour before administering the emetic agent. Milk was given to simulate a condition that is likely to exist in actual childhood ingestion cases. LEA induced prompt emesis of a relatively short duration in both the nonfasted and nonfasted, milk-treated groups. Emesis induced by Syrup of Ipecac (when given in total doses of 12 ml) was much more delayed and of much greater duration (Table V).

Throughout the testing for emetic activity, there were no signs of toxicity related to LEA or Syrup of Ipecac.

TOXICOLOGY

Doses of 5 ml/kg of LEA or Syrup of Ipecac were given to groups of two beagle dogs (1 male, 1 female) at 9:30 a.m. (Table VI).

Emesis occurred promptly in both dogs given LEA and continued intermittently for four minutes. Observations were made periodically for the rest of the day, and daily thereafter until sacrifice on the seventh day after treatment. There were no signs of toxicity observed throughout the seven day period of observation. At autopsy, the male dog appeared grossly normal; the female dog displayed signs of mild-to-moderate irritation of the gastrointestinal tract such as may be present in mild gastritis. With the exception of evidence of mild gastroenteritis, histopathology of the above dogs was unremarkable.

Administration of 5 ml/kg of Syrup of Ipecac produced emesis within 17 minutes in the male dog. Emesis did not occur until after 60 minutes in the female dog. The vomitus of both dogs became blood-tinged after repeated emetic episodes. Except for apparent fatigue, the animals appeared grossly normal upon the cessation of emesis. However, the male dog became severely depressed on the second day after treatment and died late in the afternoon of that day. Autopsy revealed widespread hemorrhage throughout the intercostal musculature, the intestinal mucosa, and the gonads. The female dog was grossly normal throughout the seven day period of observation. At autopsy, the only signs related to the treatment were mild irritation of the gastrointestinal tract.

Histopathologic examination of the male dog confirmed the observations made at autopsy, and revealed a pattern of lesions which is consistent with toxicity from ipecac--congestion of the pulmonary vessels, severe gastroenteritis with hemorrhagic lesions, and congestion, edema, and/or hemorrhage of the lymph nodes, the thymus, and the spleen. Histopathology of the female dog was unremarkable with the exception of very mild enteritis.

In addition to the above toxicologic evaluation of the emetic materials, determinations of acute oral toxicity (rats) and eye irritation (rabbits) were performed (Table VII and VIII). LEA and Syrup of Ipecac were essentially equivalent in these tests.

DISCUSSION

Physicians at poison control centers agree that the speed with which a treatment becomes effective to prevent or delay the absorption of a poison is paramount. Speed and reliability, therefore, are very important characteristics of an emetic agent that is to be used for persons who have ingested potentially hazardous materials.

As described in this report, the onset of emesis following the administration of LEA to dogs that had been pretreated with milk was more rapid than following ipecac (5 minutes vs. 25 minutes). In addition, doses of Syrup of Ipecac which had been shown to induce emesis in about 90% of the dogs tested were reduced in effectiveness to only 50% by pretreatment with the phenothiazine, chlorpromazine. Under similar conditions, the effectiveness of LEA was unaltered.

The ability of LEA to induce emesis reliably in animals pretreated with chlorpromazine may be of considerable importance. Children may be given phenothiazine-based drugs in attempts to control emesis resulting from various disturbances, to prevent itching arising from a variety of disorders, or to produce a tranquilizing effect. It is desirable to have available an emetic agent whose action is unaffected by drugs, such as the phenothiazines, which inhibit the actions of emetic agents that act through the chemoreceptor trigger zone.

It is concluded that LEA shows promise for development as a useful emetic agent in treating the ingestion of potentially hazardous materials.

TABLE I

LEA FORMULA

STP	8.0%
TKPP	12.0%
Sodium Saccharin	2.5%
Strawberry Flavoring	2 drops/30 ml
Water (distilled)	to volume

TABLE II

EFFECT OF CPZ ON LEA EMESIS

Treatment	Beagles		Emetic Means	
	Treated	Vomiting	Onset	Duration
LEA[1], no CPZ	12	10	3 min.	1 min.
LEA, plus CPZ[2]	12	12	3 min.	1 min.
Water (control)[3]	12	0	–	–

[1] Liquid Emetic Agent, 0.15 ml/kg, intragastric

[2] Chlorpromazine HCl, 2.0 mg/kg, subcutaneous

[3] Distilled water, intragastric

TABLE III

EFFECT OF CPZ ON IPECAC EMESIS

Treatment	Beagles		Emetic Means	
	Treated	Vomiting	Onset	Duration
Ipecac[1], no CPZ	12	11	38 min.	11 min.
Ipecac, plus CPZ[2]	12	6	28 min.	18 min.
Water (control)[3]	12	0	-	-

[1]Syrup of Ipecac, 0.35 ml/kg, intragastric

[2]Chlorpromazine HCl, 2.0 mg/kg, subcutaneous

[3]Distilled water, intragastric

TABLE IV

EFFECTIVENESS OF LEA IN PRESENCE OF FOOD

| Treatment | Beagles | | Emetic Means | |
	Treated	Vomiting	Onset	Duration
LEA[1], no Milk	12	12	3 min.	3 min.
Lea, plus Milk[2]	12	12	5 min.	3 min.

[1]Liquid Emetic Agent, 5 ml intragastric

[2]Whole cows milk, 240 ml intragastric

TABLE V

EFFECTIVENESS OF IPECAC IN PRESENCE OF FOOD

| Treatment | Beagles | | Emetic Means | |
	Treated	Vomiting	Onset	Duration
Ipecac[1], no Milk	12	12	17 min.	92 min.
Ipecac, plus Milk[2]	12	12	25 min.	60 min.

[1]Syrup of Ipecac, 12 ml intragastric

[2]Whole cows milk, 240 ml intragastric

TABLE VI

ACUTE ORAL TOXICITY IN BEAGLES

| Treatment | Beagles | | Emetic Means | |
	Treated	Vomiting	Onset	Duration
LEA, 5 ml/kg	2	2	(1 and 2 min.)	4 min.
Syrup of Ipecac, 5 ml/kg	2	2	(17 and 60 min.)	(4 and 5 hrs.)

TABLE VII

ACUTE ORAL TOXICITY IN RATS

Treatment	LD_{50}	95% Confidence Limits
LEA	6.0 ml/kg	5.3 – 6.9 ml/kg
Syrup of Ipecac	7.8 ml/kg	6.8 – 8.8 ml/kg

TABLE VIII

RABBIT EYE IRRITATION

Treatment	Dose	Average Maximum Score	Corneas Involved	Eyes Normal in Indicated No. of Days
LEA	0.1 ml, nonrinsed	12.0	0/3	1 in 3; 1 in 4; 1 in 7
	0.1 ml, rinsed	2.0	0/3	2 in 1; 1 in 2
Syrup of Ipecac	0.1 ml, nonrinsed	14.0	0/3	1 in 1; 1 in 2; 1 in 3
	0.1 ml, rinsed	2.0	0/3	2 in 1; 1 in 2

A CASE OF COLCHICINE POISONING
THE PHARMACOLOGICAL ROULETTE OF ADOLESCENT POISONING

Celia Viets, M.D., F.R.C.P.(C)
Medical Director, Eastern Ontario Poison Information Centre

ABSTRACT

A girl of 14 years presented at this hospital 18 hours after apparently ingesting 60 mg Colchicine tablets. The family had sought advice one hour after the initial ingestion from an Emergency Department not designated as a Poison Centre, and was reassured that there would be no problems as this girl had already vomited. This girl was extremely sick, presenting initially with severe gastroenteritis followed by prolonged marked dysphagia and severe transient bone marrow depression. Three weeks after admission this girl had almost complete alopecia.

This case will be discussed in relation to the specific aspect of Colchicine poisoning, the importance of reliable poison information, and the incidence of overdoses in teenagers.

INTRODUCTION

Colchicine poisoning has been described in the literature by various authors as causing nausea, vomiting, severe abdominal pain, dysphagia, liver damage, hypokalaemia, convulsions, hallucinations, paralytic ileus and alopecia. The maximum single dose ingested that could be found when perusing the literature was in a 14 year old Maori school girl described by Burns (1) in New Zealand in 1968. This patient took 30 mgs of Colchicine. Another case is described by Thompson (2) in the U.K. in 1963, where the patient took a single dose of 15 mgs of Colchicine. Although both these were suicidal gestures or attempts neither of these patients admitted the overdose until 8 days and 2 days respectively after the ingestion. Fatal doses have been variously recorded, many in patients already under treatment for gout, as between 7 mgs and 65 mgs of Colchicine. This paper presents a case of acute overdose of Colchicine in a 14 year old girl who took 60 mgs of Colchicine and survived, despite exhibiting most of the symptoms recorded in the literature.

A 14 year old blonde teenager took 100 tablets of 0.6 mgs of Colchicine and 20 tablets of Phenaphen No. 3 at 18:00 hrs on 13 October 1974 after an argument with her mother and boyfriend. The Colchicine was available in the home as this child's stepfather suffered from gout. Within 1 hour of ingestion of the drugs this girl had severe nausea and vomiting. The family telephoned an area hospital not designated as a Poison Centre. The parents were told by a clerk at the emergency desk that as vomiting had occurred there was no further cause for alarm.

Table 1 indicates that 100 tablets of Colchicine were ingested equivalent to 60 mgs of Colchicine. Twenty tablets of Phenaphen No. 3 Compound were also taken which represent 324 mgs of Phenobarbital, 6,500 mgs of Acetylsalicylic acid, 0.61 mgs of Hyosciamine and 600 mgs of Codeine Phosphate. During the following 18 hours after ingestion the patient continued to have profound abdominal pain, nausea and diarrhoea and arrived at the Emergency Department of the Children's Hospital of Eastern Ontario at approximately 13:00 hrs the day following the ingestion. On arrival at our Emergency Department, the girl was noted to have severe abdominal pain radiating from the umbilicus to the loin. The patient vomited green liquid, several times and had diarrhoea. At this time the patient's vital signs were stable with the exception of a mild tachycardia. The patient was noted to be generally weak and dizzy. Electrolytes, blood gases, haemogram and serum for toxicological analysis were taken immediately. The bladder was catheterised and found to be empty. An intravenous infusion of 2/3 Glucose and 1/3 Normal Saline was set up and the patient was transferred to the Intensive Care Unit of the hospital. Our initial problem was to determine whether the patient was in kidney failure or anuric from dehydration. We reviewed all the material at our Poison Centre which is extensive, but there was relatively little specific information on Colchicine other than that found in our Standard Toxicology Books. We contacted Abbott's Laboratory in Chicago, one of the distributors of Colchicine. Despite the fact that it was Thanksgiving Day in Canada and Columbus Day in the United States, the physicians at Abbott's were most helpful particularly in view of the fact that Abbott's are not the distributor of Colchicine in North America. It appeared that Colchicine was not dialyzable and so we persued the route of intensive supportive care.

Table II shows the electrolytes on admission, and 7 hours later. In view of the extreme diarrhoea and vomiting the electrolytes and blood gases were not grossly disturbed. There was evidence of mild to moderate acidosis, but this was quickly compensated for. However, low potassium levels persisted. The intake over the first 24 hours after admission was 2,130 cc.s and the output 406 cc.s. This indicates that the patient was dehydrated. Urine was obtained approximately 1 hour after the intravenous infusion was set up.

Table III shows serial potassium levels for a week after the ingestion of Colchicine. As documented in the literature, our patient continued to have hypokalaemia despite continuous addition of potassium into the intravenous infusion. This situation persisted until the eighth day after ingestion.

Table IV shows the constituents of Phenaphen detected over the first 24 hours after admission. As the maximum level of salicylate was 15.9 mgs % it must be assumed that the patient must have vomited the Phenaphen shortly after ingestion. Codeine was negative in the blood; unfortunately urine was not sent for codeine analysis at this time.

It was not possible to analyze Colchicine locally so samples of serum and urine were frozen until we could arrange for this analysis. As Colchicine analysis is not a frequent request in the laboratory where these levels were determined, the Biochemist was not satisfied with these results. They were done by Gas Liquid Chromatography and more recently this particular laboratory has acquired a Mass Spectrometer which their Chief Biochemist felt would have produced more accurate results. The samples sent had to be pooled for the first 3 days and the next 2 days respectively as inadequate serum was available for daily determinations (Table V). However; it is of interest that the levels decreased over the first 8 days to a level of 0.9 mgs %. This decrease in serum level of Colchicine was compatible with the patient's clinical state.

The patient's blood indices were monitored daily in view of the anticipated bone marrow depression.

Table VI shows serial haematology results, but abnormal indices only are included. The haemogram on admission, that is twenty-four hours after in-gestion, indicated degeneration of polymorphs on the peripheral smear. As noted on the slide the platelets started dropping to a level of 87,000 on the fourth day and on the fifth day this level was 35,000 at which time a mild epistaxis occurred. The patient was placed on intravenous Ampicillin and isolated. The epistaxis continued intermittently over the next two days but the haemoglobin remained adequate. It is interesting to note that the haemoglobin remained at a reasonable level throughout the period of Pancytopaenia. The Platelets and White Cell Count were at their lowest on the 6th day post ingestion when the reticulocyte count was 0.1%. On the 7th day there were no reticulocytes. Gradually the White Cell Count and Platelet Count increased so that on the 10th day post ingestion the White Cell Count was normal and the Platelet Count was considered to be adequate. On the 7th day a bone marrow was performed.

Table VII shows the bone marrow findings. The bone marrow was generally hypocellular with a marked decrease in the neutrophile and erythroid series. A fragment of bone marrow was sent to the cyto genetics laboratory and 3 cells were found arrested in the metaphase state. This was considered to be an abnormal finding attributable to the effect of Colchicine on the bone marrow in vivo. No abnormal figures or breaks of the chromosomes of these 3 cells were detected.

Throughout the 10 days this patient was kept in the hospital's Intensive Care Unit, the patient continued to complain of abdominal cramp with and without diarrhoea. Intravenous infusion was maintained and the patient's symptoms were relieved by drugs on a symptomatic basis.

Table VIII shows liver function tests and serum amylase levels over a period of 3 weeks. The raised S.G.O.T. and bilirubin levels indicate liver damage and the raised amylase levels are compatible with enteritis. These factors are presumably due to the antimitotic effect of Colchicine and are confirmed by Stemmermann (3) in his autopsy findings in Human Pathology in 1971 where 3 patients suffering from

gout died after intravenous infusions of Colchicine.
The bottom half of this table indicates complete
resolution of these abnormal findings in our patient,
as the patient was re-admitted for a second overdose
of aspirin in April 1975. The amount of aspirin
taken at this admission was insignificant. However,
it did give us the opportunity of rechecking her
liver enzymes and also her blood indices both of
which were normal.

On the eighth day after ingestion of Colchicine the
patient complained of extreme abdominal pain. Flat
Plate X-Rays were taken of the abdomen and the surgeons
confirmed the findings of a toxic paralytic ileus.
The X-Rays indicated fluid levels in the colon con-
firming this diagnosis. The patient was placed on
continuous nasogastric suction. The ileus resolved
over the next 3 days. Paralytic Ileus secondary to
Colchicine taken by 2 patients suffering from gout
was documented by Moise (4) in 1965.

Our patient remained relatively well until the 13th
and 14th day when she began hallucinating at night.
The latter responded to sedation and reassurance.

On the 17th hospital day, the patient who was admitted with thick natural blonde hair began losing
her hair. At the time of discharge the patient had
lost 90% of her hair and later became totally
alopeicic for a total of approximately 10 weeks. Six
months after the original ingestion of Colchicine
this patient, as already mentioned, was re-admitted
to the hospital with a second overdose. At the time
of her re-admission in April 1975, the hair had re-
grown approximately 3 inches in length but was dark
and no longer blonde. Burns (1) referred to
alopecia in his Maori girl and Thompson (2) in 1963
refers to alopecia in an 18 year old boy who took
an overdose of Colchicine. Brown (5) makes reference
to the fact that blondes are most susceptible to

alopecia from Colchicine. This would seem to be the case in our patient as the alopecia was more profound and prolonged than in the other cases described.

When this patient had made adequate recovery she stated that she would not have taken the tablets if she knew that they would have made her so sick, and admitted that the tablets were taken because of the chaos of her home. As noted 6 months later she once more resorted to a manipulative suicide gesture as plans were being made to send her to a treatment home. This overdose consisted of a very few aspirins, hence the pharmacological roulette of teenage poisoning. In 1972 when our Poison Information Centre was situated in a 1,000 bed general hospital we treated 737 patients for self-poisoning and 162 were teenagers. In view of the shortage of beds only severely poisoned patients were generally admitted. In 1972 we admitted 250 patients. Careful review of these admitted self-poisoned patients indicated a peak incidence in teenagers and young adults between twenty and twenty-four years. The highest incidence of repeat overdoses in our admitted patients in 1972 was noted to be in teenagers. Kessel (6) also made note in his study on self-poisoning in 1965 that the highest incidence of self-poisoning occurred in teenagers and young adults.

In summary a case of Colchicine overdose is presented where the patient developed severe gastro-enteritis with abdominal pain, persistant hypokalaemia, a toxic ileus, pancytopaenia with epistaxis, liver damage, hallucinations and complete alopecia. All symptoms were resolved when the patient was re-admitted 6 months later, with the exception of the patient's unstable personality. This patient taking 60 mgs of Colchicine in a single dose, took, as far as is known, the largest single dose recorded in the literature and survived. It is suggested that if the parents had contacted a well organized Poison

Information Centre initially many of this patient's symptoms could have been avoided. Brief reference is made to a year's experience with self-poisoning in a large general hospital in 1972. Particular note is made of the high incidence of self-poisoning in teenagers.

REFERENCES

1. Burns BJ: Colchicine toxicity. *Australasian Annals of Medicine* 17:341, 1968.

2. Thompson GW: Alopecia totalis following suicidal colchicine overdose. *J Royal Army Cps* 110:113, 1964.

3. Stemmermann GN, Hayashi T: Colchicine toxicity, *Human Pathology* 2:321, 1971.

4. Moise R, Asch L, Wiederkehr JL: Ileus Paralytique apres colchicotherapie. *Semaine des Hospitaux* 41:1030, Paris, 1965.

5. Brown WO, Seed L: Effect of colchicine on human tissues. *Amer J Clin Pathol* 15:189, 1945.

6. Kessel N: Self poisoning, Part 1. *Brit Med J* 2:1265-1270, 1965.

TABLE I

DRUGS INGESTED 1800 HRS 13.10.74

COLCHICINE TABS 0.6 mgs x 100 = 60 mgs

PHENAPHEN TABS x 20 = (PHENOBARBITAL 16.2 mgx x 20 = 324 mgs
No. 3

(A.S.A. 325 mgs x 20 = 6500 mgs

(HYOSCIAMINE 0.031 mgs x 20 = 0.61 mgs

(CODEINE PHOSPHATE 30 mgs x 20 = 600 mgs

13.10.74   1900 HRS TELEPHONE ADVICE GIVEN FROM ANOTHER AREA
HOSPITAL

14.10.74   1315 HRS PATIENT ARRIVED AT C.H.E.O.* EMERGENCY AND
ADMITTED

* = CHILDREN'S HOSPITAL OF EASTERN ONTARIO

TABLE II

ELECTROLYTE STATUS ON ADMISSION 14.10.74

	1410 HRS	2100 HRS
B.U.N.	10 mgs%	8 mgs%
Na	146 meq/l	140 meq/l
K.	3.3 meq/l	2.6 meq/l
pH	7.45	7.33
PCO_2	25 mmHg	26 mmHg
PO_2	55 mmHg	82 mmHg
B/Excess	-3.8 meq/l	-10 meq/l
HCO_3	17 meq/l	14 meq/l
$T.CO_2$	18 mM/l	15 mM/l

INGESTION OF COLCHICINE 13.10.74 1800 HRS

TABLE III

SERIAL POTASSIUM LEVELS

14.10.74	1410 HRS	3.3 meq/l
14.10.74	1730 HRS	2.6 meq/l
14.10.74	2100 HRS	2.7 meq/l
15.10.74	355 HRS	3.0 meq/l
15.10.74	P.M.	3.1 meq/l
16.10.74		3.4 meq/l
17.10.74		3.8 meq/l
18.10.74		3.6 meq/l
19.10.74		4.5 meq/l

INGESTION OF COLCHICINE 13.10.74   1800 HRS

TABLE IV

TOXICOLOGY LEVELS

PHENAPHEN

14.10.74	1410 HRS	PHENOBARBITONE	POSITIVE
		SALICYLATE	11 mgs%
		CODEINE	Not present
	1730 HRS	SALICYLATE	15.9 mgs%
15.10.74	355 HRS	SALICYLATE	15.4 mgs%

TABLE V

TOXICOLOGY LEVELS

COLCHICINE

14.10.74)

15.10.74) POOLED SERUM LEVEL COLCHICINE ▬ 5 mgs%

16.10.74)

17.10.74)
                POOLED SERUM LEVEL COLCHICINE = 2.3 mgs%
18.10.74)

22.10.74   SINGLE SERUM LEVEL COLCHICINE = 0.9 mg%

15.10.74   SINGLE URINE SAMPLE NEGATIVE FOR COLCHICINE

TABLE VI

HAEMATOLOGY RESULTS   POST-INGESTION

	WBC x 10^3	HGB.Gm		PLATELETS	RETICULOCYTES
DAY 2	7.4	11.5		475,000	
DAY 3	22.3	13.6		190,000	
DAY 4	9.2	11.8		87,000	
DAY 5	3.2	10.6		35,000*	
DAY 6	2.8	10.7	Approx.	19,000	0.1%
DAY 7	3.5	11.9		48,000**	0.0%
DAY 8	6.0	11.9		122,000	0.1%
DAY 9	8.5	12.0		191,000	1.0%
DAY 10	7.6	12.2		300,000	1.6%
DAY 11	8.6	11.8		Adequate	

*   PATIENT ISOLATED

**   BONE MARROW FOR MORPHOLOGY AND CYTOGENETICS

TABLE VII

BONE MARROW FINDINGS DAY 7

BLASTS	1%	LYMPHOCYTES	35%
PROMYELOCYTE	4%	PLASMA CELLS	2%
MYELOCTYE	10%	RETICULAR CELLS	3%
METAMYELOCYTE	8%	MONOCYTES	5%
BANDS	8%	PRO-ERYTHROBLASTS	0%
POLYS	7%	ERYTHROBLASTS	1%
EOSINOPHILS	6%	NORMOBLASTS	8%

MARROW FRAGMENTS ALL HYPOCELLULAR

TABLE VIII

LIVER FUNCTION TESTS   AMYLASE LEVELS

	S.G.O.T.	TOTAL BILIRUBIN	AMYLASE
17.10.74	358 I.U./litre	1.1 mgs/dl	250 I.U./litre
24.10.74	103 I.U./litre	2.3 mgs/dl	540 I.U./litre
29.10.74			525 I.U./litre
31.10.74	165 I.U./litre	0.6 mgs/dl	165 I.U./litre
06.11.74	61 I.U./litre		271 I.U./litre

ALKALINE PHOSPHATASE LEVELS NORMAL

RE-ADMISSION 07.04.75 (for A.S.A. Overdose)

S.G.O.T. = 20   Total Bilirubin less than 1 mg.

DIAGNOSIS AND MANAGEMENT OF COMA DUE TO EXOGENOUS TOXINS

Howard C. Mofenson, M.D., F.A.A.P.
Director, Poison Control Center, Nassau County
Medical Center, New York
Professor of Clinical Pediatrics, State University
of New York at Stony Brook

Joseph Greensher, M.D., F.A.A.P.
Associate Director, Poison Control Center, Nassau
County Medical Center, New York
Associate Professor of Clinical Pediatrics, State
University of New York at Stony Brook

ABSTRACT

The patient brought to the emergency room in coma which is not readily explained by history or physical examination is most frequently suffering from a suicide attempt, drug abuse or accidental poisoning.

The emergency treatment of coma should proceed concurrently with attempts at differential diagnosis.

This presentation discusses the emergency management of the comatose patient, differentiates neurologic-structural from toxic-metabolic coma, and further separates metabolic from exogenous coma. Clinical clues and bedside diagnostic tests are presented to aid the clinician in defining a precise etiologic agent.

The nontoxic ingestions are not true poisonings and can be adequately handled with simple reassurance by a poison information center or a knowledgeable physician. A nontoxic ingestion is the consumption of a nonedible product which usually does not produce symptoms. No product or drug is entirely safe, all

can produce undesireable effects if ingested in sufficiently great concentration or amount.

The knowledge of the nontoxic ingestion serves to
avoid overtreatment, placing the victim in jeopardy
of a panicky automobile ride to the physician or the
nearest medical facility, and serves as a warning of
inadequate supervision or improper and unsafe environment and the potential of future, more serious ingestions. This knowledge allows us to recommend the
least toxic product to do the job for use in the home.

The designation of the "nontoxic ingestion" requires
the following criteria:

1. Absolute identification of the product.
2. Absolute assurance that only a single product
   was ingested.
3. Assurance that there is no signal word on the
   container.
4. A good approximation of the amount ingested.
5. Assurance that the victim is free of symptoms.
6. The ability to call back at intervals to
   determine that no symptoms have developed.

The designation of a nontoxic ingestion requires
exact historical data of the incident, and product
identification. The information obtained should allow
the questioner to feel confident that other products,
besides the designated one, have not been ingested
and reasonable certainty as to the amount ingested.
The volume of a swallow of $1\frac{1}{2}$ - 3 year old child is
4.5 cc, and adult is 15 cc. This may allow an estimation of the amount ingested when the ingestion has
been observed. The designation of a large amount is
difficult to define.

A good rule of thumb for the toxicity of the average
drug is that five times the therapeutic dose may be a
toxic dose. A documented single tablet of medication
even in adult dosage will not produce significant

toxicity if ingested by a child. Opiate narcotics are the exception; an ingestion of opiate narcotics requires medical examination and careful observation because of the narrow margin of safety, especially with Lomotil (Diphenyoxalate).

The emetic property of the ingested substance is important. Rodents do not vomit, therefore, the rodent LD50 is invalid when the defense mechanism in humans and other animals is overlooked. In detergents (anionic phosphate type) if emesis has not been induced by the toxic agent it is unlikely that a systemic toxic dose has been ingested.

The type of packaging may aid in determining whether a toxic amount could have been ingested - spray aersol containers, pump containers, squeeze tubes, etc. rarely will produce a toxic ingestion.

The label and signal word is a clue to the toxicity of the product. If it states "Danger Poison", has an antidote statement or states "Call Physician Immediately" on the label, it is extremely toxic. Any label on the container "Danger Poison", "Warning", "Caution", automatically removes the product from the category of a nontoxic ingestion. The label "Keep Out of Reach of Children" has no significance since many products with minimal toxicity carry this label.

Any symptom, even if it appears unrelated to the ingestion, should exclude the diagnosis of a nontoxic ingestion without a medical examination.

In 1976 the Nassau County Medical Center received 6,256 reports of ingestion of nonedible products by children under five years of age. Only 253 had to be examined in the emergency room and only 48 required hospitalization. On the basis of telephone information the Center was able to designate 641 of these calls as nontoxic and requiring no therapy except for reassurance.

The six years that have elapsed since our original
tabulation in 1970 have allowed us to add many products
to our original list of nontoxic ingestions.

Table I represents frequently ingested products that
are usually nontoxic.

Plant identification is very difficult, but if the
caller can identify the plant and if it is listed in
the non-toxic list below (Table II), we advise simple
observation.

Children over the age of 5 years should be excluded
from consideration as a nontoxic ingestion. Ingestions
by these children may indicate an intolerable home
situation that requires medical and psychiatric evaluation. These ingestions are often a "cry for help".

TABLE I

FREQUENTLY INGESTED PRODUCTS THAT ARE USUALLY NONTOXIC

Abrasives
Adhesives
Antacides*
Antibiotics
Baby Product Cosmetics*
Ballpoint Pen Inks
Bathtub Floating Toys
Battery (Dry Cell) (1/5 MLD of
  Mercuric Chloride)
Bath Oil (Castor Oil & Perfume)*
Bleach (Less than 5% Sodium Hypochlorite)*
Body Conditioners*
Bubble Bath Soaps (Detergents)
Calamine Lotion*
Candles (Beeswax or paraffin)
Caps (toy pistols) (potassium chlorate)
Chalk (calcium carbonate)
Cigarettes or Cigars (Nicotine)
Clay (modeling)
Colognes
Contraceptive Pills
Corticosteroids*
Cosmetics*
Crayons (marked A.P., C.P.)
Dehumidifying Packets (Silica or Charcoal)
Detergents (Phosphate)
Deodorants
Deodorizers (spray and refrigerator)
Elmer's Glue*
Etch-A-sketch*
Eye Makeup*
Fabric Softeners*
Fertilizer (If no insecticides or
  Herbicides added)*
Fish Bowl Additives
Glues & Pastes*
Golf Ball (core may cause mechanical
  injury)
Grease*
Hair Products (Dyes, sprays, tonics)*
Hand Lotions and Creams*
Hydrogen Peroxide (Medicinal 3%)*
Incense*
Indelible Markers
Ink (Black, Blue)
Iodophil Disinfectant*
Laxatives*

Lipstick*
Lubricant*
Lubricating Oils*
Lysol Brand Disinfectant (Not Toilet
  Bowl Cleaner)*
Magic Markers
Makeup (Eye, Liquid Facial)*
Matches
Mineral Oil*
Newspaper*
Paint - Indoor - Latex
Pencil (Lead-graphite, coloring)
Perfumes
Petroleum Jelly (Vaseline)
Phenolphthalein Laxatives (Ex-Lax)*
Play-Doh
Polaroid Picture Coating Fluid
Porous-tip ink marking pens
Prussian Blue (Fericyanide)*
Putty (less than 2 oz.)
Rough*
Rubber Cement*
Sachets (Essential Oils, Powder)
Shampoos (Liquid)
Shaving Creams and Lotions
Soap and Soap Products
Spackles*
Suntan Preparation*
Sweetening Agents (Saccharin, Cyclamates)
Teething Rings (Water-sterility?)
Thermometers (Mercury)
Thyroid Tablet*
Toilet Water*
Tooth Paste (with and without Fluoride)
Vaseline*
Vitamins - with or without Fluoride
Warfarin*
Water Colors*
Zinc Oxide*
Zirconium Oxide*

The average swallow of a child
under 5 years of age is 5 ml.
The average adult swallow is 15 ml.

*Indicates new additions to the list of nontoxic ingestions.

TABLE II

NON-TOXIC HOUSE PLANTS*

African Violet (Saintpaulia Sonantha)
Aralia False (Dizygotheca Elegantissima)
Begonia (Botanical Name)
Boston Fern (Nephrolepis Exata)
Christmas Cactus (Zygocactus Truncactus)
Coleus (Botanical Name)
Creeping Charlie (Pilea Nummularifolia or
     Plectranthus Austalis)
Donkey Tail (Sedum Morganianum)
Dracaena (Species)
Hawaiian Ti (Cordyline Terminalis)
Hen & Chicks (Escheveria or Sempervivum Tectorus)
Hoya-Botanical Name (Wax Plant)
Jade Plant (Crassula Argentea)
Lipstick Plant (Aeschynanthus Lobbianus)
Mother-in-Law Tongue (Sanservieria Trifasciata)
Monkey Plant (Ruella Makoyana)
Peperomia (Botanical Name)
Piggy-Back Plant (Tolmiea Menziestii)
Pilea (Botanical Name)
Pink Polka Dot Plant (Hypoestes Sanguinolenta)
Plectranthus (Botanical Name)
Prayer Plant (Maranta Leuconeura Kerchoveana)
Rosary Bean Plant (Ceropegia Woodii)
Rosary Pearls (Senico Rowleyanus or S. Herreianus)
Rubber Plant (Ficus Elastica)
Schefflera (Brassaia Actinophylla)
Sensitive Plant (Mimosa Pudica)
Spider Plant (Anthericum or Chlorophytum Cosmosum)
Swedish Ivy (Plectranthus Australis)
Wandering Jew (Zebrina Pendula)
Weeping Fig (Ficus Benjamina)

*Taken from the Poison Information Newsletter, Mary
Bridge Children's Health Center.

ANALYSES OF COMMUNITY AWARENESS PRIOR TO POISON
PREVENTION EDUCATION PROGRAM

Virginia Hartline
*Poison Prevention Council of Kalamazoo,
Kalamazoo, Michigan   49006*

ABSTRACT

   *Poisoning is the leading cause of accidental death
in children under five years of age. The Poison
Prevention Council of Kalamazoo (PPCK) was established
in the fall of 1975 to educate the public about
poisonous materials and to increase the awareness of
procedures to be taken in the event poisoning should
occur. A preliminary study to determine public awareness before the institution of the Kalamazoo Poison
Prevention Program is described.*

   *The names of all women having delivered babies in
Kalamazoo in 1973 were obtained from the birth records
on file in the county courthouse. The year 1973 was
chosen realizing these children to be in the highest
risk group for poisoning in the current year. Each
woman was contacted by telephone and asked for information concerning the ingestion of poisonous substances
by their children in instances when assistance from a
physician or a poison control center was obtained.
The poisonous agent and age of the child were noted.
Information was also gathered concerning the availability, knowledge, and use of syrup of ipecac.*

   *At this time 324 women have been reached; 68
poison ingestions have been documented. 58.1% of
those contacted have ipecac in their homes at the
present time, but 30% of the sample were totally
unaware of ipecac and its use. The PPCK is presently
engaged in outreach programs directed at new mothers,*

*school children, and the general public. This
evaluation will be repeated in the future to determine
the impact of the PPCK program on public awareness of
poison prevention methods and upon the incidence of
poisonings among children following the implementation of this program.*

INTRODUCTION

Nine townships covering 576 square miles comprise
the urban center of southwestern Michigan known as
Kalamazoo County. Kalamazoo centers a 6 county
trading area equidistant from Detroit and Chicago.
The 200,000 plus population is composed of 80% native
born American citizens. The majority of naturalized
citizens come from the Netherlands. More than 25 of
the largest corporations in the United States have
established plant operations in the county. Three
colleges and a large university provide cultural,
athletic and educational advantages to the Kalamazoo
community. The families of this community comprised
the study group used for the analysis of poison awareness which began in the fall of 1975.

The originators of the Poison Prevention Council in
Kalamazoo were familiar with a similar organization
working in the Detroit area. Upon transferring to
Kalamazoo, inquiries were made as to the need for
such an organization in southwestern Michigan. The
idea of a women's interest group concerned with disseminating information on behalf of the poison control
centers was enthusiastically received.

The Poison Prevention Council of Kalamazoo became
effective on June 17, 1975, with the expanded purpose
of educating the public about poisonous materials and
increasing the awareness of procedures to be taken in
the event poisoning should occur. The organization
is composed of 25 women of varying backgrounds. It
is locally funded, receiving no State or Federal aid.

The P.P.C. works in conjunction with 4 other counties comprising the Great Lakes Poison Information Network.

As organization began on the Council's program for the year, it appeared beneficial to estimate the sophistication of the community's awareness before beginning an intensive educational schedule. Thus, the ability to evaluate the benefit to the community would be available in years to come.

There are approximately 3,000 babies born in the two local Kalamazoo hospitals each year. The year 1973 was chosen for this study, realizing these children to be in the highest risk group for poisoning in the current year. The purpose of this study was not only to collect data from the Kalamazoo area, but also to increase public awarenss to the possibility of poisoning and the availability of help in such an incident.

METHOD

The names of all women living in Kalamazoo County having delivered babies in 1973 were obtained from birth records on file in the County Clerk's Office. This group will henceforth be called the "total maternal population." The following data was noted: mother's name, father's name, mother's age in 1973 and family address. Telephone numbers were obtained from the current Kalamazoo telephone directory. Families contacted comprised the study group. The maternal age distribution of the study group compared to the total maternal population was used as an index of the reliability of the study. Each family contacted by telephone was asked for information concerning the ingestion of poisonous substances by their children in instances when assistance from a physician or poison control center was obtained. The poisonous agent and age of the child were noted. Information was also gathered concerning the availability, knowledge and use of Syrup of Ipecac.

RESULTS

The total maternal population in 1973 in Kalamazoo County was 2,217. Telephone numbers were obtained for 1,091 of these families. Two hundred and ninety-two families were unable to be reached by telephone. The loss of 268 families was attributed to change of telephone number since the publication of the most recent directory, divorce or relocation. Twenty-four of these calls were discontinued after 5 separate attempts at reaching these families. Five women refused to participate in the study. The study population consisted of 794 families.

Table I shows the maternal Age Distribution of the total population as compared to the study group. The discrepancy in the data obtained on the younger aged mothers is attributed to the transience of this age family between the years of 1973-1975. The sizable student population in Kalamazoo may be a significant contributing factor in the lack of data obtained in the less than 18 to 21 maternal age group.

Within the study group population of 794 families, 118 families experienced 1 poison ingestion involving 1 child. Four families experienced 1 episode of poisoning involving more than 1 child in the family. Ten cases of poisoning resulted this way. Fourteen families experienced 2 separate poisoning incidents resulting in 28 children ingesting toxic substances. One hundred and fifty-six poisonings were recorded. Seventeen percent of the families contacted had a recorded poison ingestion. Five percent of the families contacted experienced 2 separate poisoning incidents.

Table II shows the age distribution of childhood poison ingestions recorded. Of the poisoning incidents recorded, 96% occurred in children under 5 years of age, 79% occurred between the ages of 1 and 3.

Table III shows the analysis of the ingested substances. Forty-seven percent of all substances ingested were oral medications. There were 19 ingestions of aspirin or aspirin containing drugs. Children's chewable vitamins accounted for 17 of the medicinal ingestions. In the category classified as hydrocarbons, paint thinner accounted for 6 of the 14 poisonings.

In analyzing the maternal age distribution among families in which poisoning occurred, these results shown in Table IV were obtained. Except for the 30-32 age group, the incidence of poisonings did not vary with maternal age. The increased incidence of poisoning within the 30-32 age group of 25% was statistically significant (p<0.05).

An analysis of the data collected on the knowledge and use of Ipecac showed that 72% of the study population knew of Ipecac and its use. Of this knowledgeable 72%, 83% had Ipecac in their home at the time of contact. Sixty percent of the total study group had Ipecac in their home. Twenty-eight percent of the study group were totally unaware of Ipecac and its use.

Table V shows the percentage of women at varying ages who had no knowledge of Ipecac. The 63% of women in the 18-20 age group having no knowledge of Ipecac as contrasted with 28% in the entire study group is statistically significant (p<0.001).

When analyzed by maternal age (Table VI), it is noted that only 67% of mothers between 18-20 years of age who were knowledgeable about the drug and its use had Ipecac in the home. This age group was the least knowledgeable of Ipecac and when the awareness was apparent, they were the least likely to have Ipecac in the home.

Of the 14 families where more than 1 incidence of poison ingestion occurred, 36% had no Ipecac although all were familiar with the drug and its use.

Experience with a poisoning episode increased a family's knowledge of Ipecac. Within the families where poisoning occurred, 90% showed awareness of the drug in comparison to 72% in the study population as a whole. But this experience with poison ingestion did not lead to a greater percentage likelihood (83 to 88%) that a family would have Ipecac in their home. However, a poisoning incident did increase the overall chance that Ipecac would be found in the home.

CONCLUSION

The educational program of the Kalamazoo Poison Prevention Council focuses its attention on kindergarten and nursery school children, young mothers and young girls of babysitting age.

The data obtained in this study confirms that most poisonings occur between the ages of 1 and 3. This child is very difficult to reach from an educational standpoint. The group therefore concentrated its effort on kindergarten and nursery school children (not at high risk for poisoning, themselves). The use of a puppet show demonstrating the dangers of poisonous materials was thought to be a successful means of impressing this age group. These children were encouraged to initiate poison patrols to eliminate dangerous substances from areas inhabited by younger children in the home. This age child is enthusiastic toward his role as helper in the home.

The most common substances ingested by children were oral medications. The puppet show used by the Kalamazoo Poison Prevention Council expressly explains the proper use of medications and the danger involved in abuse.

It was noted in the data collected on the awareness and use of Ipecac that the 18-20 year old mother has the least amount of knowledge concerning the drug and is most unlikely to have it in the home. Programs encouraging poison prevention might be appropriate for teenagers either within the school or special interest groups such as the Girl Scouts which would increase awareness before a young mother is faced with a poison ingestion she cannot handle. Pre-natal or post-natal education classes might also be used to disseminate this information.

A poisoning episode increased parental knowledge to the use and effectiveness of Ipecac, however, these families were no more likely to have Ipecac in the home than the total population. Physicians and emergency room personnel might encourage appropriation of Ipecac at the time of treatment for poison ingestion.

During the telephone contact made to the 794 families, all parents were advised to call their physician or the Poison Control Center before using Ipecac and all were given the Hot Line number of the Poison Control Center.

With this baseline data obtained from the study, assessment regarding the awareness of Ipecac can be used in the future.

TABLE I

MATERNAL AGE DISTRIBUTION

Maternal Age	Total Maternal Population	Study Population
<18	3%	9%
18-20	14%	7%
21-23	23%	18%
24-26	24%	30%
27-29	17%	21%
30-32	10%	13%
33-35	4%	5%
36-38	2%	3%
39-41	9%	3%
>41	4%	2%
Unknown	10%	3%

TABLE II

AGE DISTRIBUTION OF CHILDHOOD POISON INGESTIONS

Age of Child	Number of Children	% of Poisoned Population	Cumulative %
<1	3	2%	2
1	47	30%	32
2	74	47%	79
3	15	10%	89
4	7	4%	93
5	5	3%	96
6	1	0.6%	96.6
>6	0		
Unknown	4	3%	99.6

TABLE III

SUBSTANCES INVOLVED IN 156 CHILD POISONINGS

	Number	%
Drugs & Medications:	74	47%
Aspirin & Aspirin cont. drugs - 19		
Vitamins 17		
Cough, cold, allergy med. - 12		
Topical Med. 7		
Miscellaneous 19		
Household Products:	19	12%
Cosmetics:	15	10%
Plants:	13	8%
Hydrocarbons:	14	9%
Paint Thinner - 6		
Kerosene - 3		
Furn. Polish - 2		
Miscellaneous - 3		
Miscellaneous:	16	10%
Unknown:	5	3%

TABLE IV

MATERNAL AGE DISTRIBUTION IN FAMILIES WHERE POISONING OCCURRED

Maternal Age	Number of Mothers	Number of Poisonings	%
<18	7	1	14%
18-20	59	8	14%
21-23	139	19	14%
24-26	241	42	17%
27-29	165	27	16%
30-32	103	26	25%*
33-35	39	6	15%
36-38	20	3	15%
39-41	9	1	11%
>41	5	0	
		133	

*p<0.05

TABLE V

Maternal Age	% Having No Knowledge
<18	43
18-20	63*
21-23	32
24-26	24
27-29	19
30-32	19
33-35	36
36-38	35
39-41	11
>41	60
All	28%

TABLE VI

Maternal Age	Know	&	Have
<18	4		100
18-20	14		67
21-23	75		80
24-26	150		83
27-29	117		87
30-32	69		83
33-35	23		92
36-38	11		85
39-41	7		88
>41	2		100

AN EVALUATION OF COMMUNITY MEDICAL SERVICES: THE
MARYLAND POISON INFORMATION CENTER MASS MEDIA CAMPAIGN

Gary Oderda, Pharm.D.
*Assistant Professor of Clinical Pharmacy and Director,
Maryland Poison Information Center, University of
Maryland School of Pharmacy*

Arlene Fonaroff, M.P.H., Ph.D.
*Staff Officer, Assembly on Behavioral and Social
Sciences, National Academy of Sciences
Associate Professorial Lecturer in Epidemiology and
Environmental Health, George Washington University*

ABSTRACT

   *This paper reports results of a public mass media
campaign to convey information on a regional poison
center. A baseline measure was established through
a random sample telephone survey (N=200) in the catch-
ment area to determine emergency service systems known
and used by laypeople in post-ingestion periods. After
8 months a second random sample of the same size, in
the same area, was contacted. The before-after study
evaluates public knowledge of how to reach and use
poison emergency services. It reveals differences in
emergency action taken on ingestion of a poisonous
substance, including data on access and use of the
poison information center, physician, ambulance and
emergency services. The study demonstrates effectiveness of mass media in providing useable information
for public action in post-ingestion periods. Indication of cost factors in emergency action are provided.*

   *In the pre-test, 12% of respondents said they would
call the poison center if faced with an ingestion.
This increased to 14.5% in the post-test. A significant increase was seen in the number of respondents in
the post-test who knew the poison center phone number*

*or had ready access to it. Of the 200 respondents in
the post-test, 121 (60.5%) knew who Mr. Yuk was and
could state his purpose.*

Background and Purpose of Study

The control of injury caused by ingestion of liquid
and solid substances found in the residential or occupational environments is a major public health problem. If we view the phenomena of poisonous ingestions
as a system in which products are perceived as needed,
secured, stored, used and then stored again for future
use, intervening variables show themselves in the form
of actions which may be altered at three points in the
system: before the injury occurs, by either totally
eliminating or controlling availability and access to
potentially hazardous substances; during the injury
event itself, by controlling the type and amount of
substance ingested; and after the injury, by such
action as early detection, treatment or other remedial
acts (1). It is readily apparent that events before,
during, and after injury may be managed through behavioral choice of the individual or through environmental
designs and controls (2).

This paper focuses on environmental control of poison
ingestions in the pre and post-injury periods. Environmental control will be examined through the functions
assumed by an organized component of a community medical
emergency service network, the poison information center
(PIC). Specifically, we will examine effectiveness of
a public education function designed to increase public
awareness of PIC services and how they may be obtained.

Poison Centers exist to alter morbidity and mortality
attributed to ingestion of poisonous substances. Their
role is to increase public awareness of hazardous substances in the residential environment which may result
in poisoning on ingestion; to inform the public of a

In addition to NCPCC, there are several other organizations serving as clearinghouses of current data on product toxicity and treatment measures. One such group is the National Poison Center Network, with central offices in Pittsburgh, PA. A unique service offered by this network is a mass media public education program.

While many state and local poison information centers actively engage in public education about poison prevention and PIC service, it is often overlooked as an integral part of a community's emergency medical care service system. This paper reports results of a study concerned with the extent to which a state supported center, the Maryland Poison Information Center (MPIC), succeeded in providing public information about its services through use of the television package program developed by the National Poison Center Network. The evaluation is based on knowledge disseminated to the public primarily through use of four television spot announcements. In order to identify differences in emergency action taken in the event of poisonous substance ingestion, data were collected on public access to and use of home remedies, the MPIC, the physician, ambulance and emergency hospital services.

MPIC Efforts to Increase Public Awareness

The MPIC is a division of the University of Maryland School of Pharmacy. Inquiries involving poisoning are received from both the general public and health professionals. MPIC has no treatment facilities; all information is provided by telephone. Individuals in need of emergency treatment are referred directly to local treatment facilities. Phone calls received by MPIC include reports of human and animal ingestions; inquiries about drug use, drug interactions, and other medical information. A call is recorded as an ingestion when a human is exposed to a substance (drug, chemical or household product), toxic or non-toxic, by

24-hour telephone service which provides directions
for the lay public on what to do if a potentially
poisonous substance is ingested; to recommend treatment for reported cases involving the ingestion of
household products and medicines to the medical community; to provide comprehensive information to the
medical community on ingredients, toxicity, expected
signs and symptoms; and to collect ingestion data for
epidemiological analysis.

While originally developed to assist the professional
community, by 1968 an estimated 75% of all telephone
inquiries came from laypeople who had learned of the
24-hour telephone emergency service provided by poison
information centers (3).

In 1957, a National Clearinghouse for Poison Control
Centers (NCPCC) was established to coordinate activities of individual centers, to provide them with data
on poisoning topics; and to collate the annual statistics voluntarily contributed by centers on epidemiological aspects of poisonings. In 1974, 580 centers
were part of the NCPCC, 540 of them regularly submit-
ting ingestion reports to NCPCC. The epidemiology of
poison ingestions in the United States is derived from
these data (4). The NCPCC data is limited further in
that many large regional poison centers do not submit
their ingestion data to this clearinghouse. It is
important to note that this epidemiological profile is
believed to represent less than 15% of true incidence.

In 1972, NCPCC reported that approximately 161,000
Americans were injured through ingesting poisonous
substances and that approximately 48% of this group
received some form of medical treatment. The dimen-
sions of the problem are even more startling in that
an estimated 65% of total reported ingestions refer to
children under 5 years of age, and that the ingestion
of poisonous substances is one of the five leading
causes of death in ages 0-4 (5).

any route (oral, topical, etc.) (6).

Mass media serves as the primary means to inform the public about the MPIC. Information presented includes the center's phone number and the kinds of services provided. In 1974, the MPIC obtained a state wide toll-free number which is printed with all other emergency call numbers on the front inside cover of all but one of the telephone directories in the State of Maryland.

Since its inception in 1966, when the center received 1,531 telephone calls, use of its services has steadily increased. A record number of phone inquiries (16,726) was reported in 1974, coinciding with the installation of the state-wide toll-free number. Using the 1974 data, the nature of MPIC calls are summarized below (7). These data parallel trends throughout the United States.

1. 84% of total human ingestion calls (11,763 or 13,989) were from laypeople seeking advice on poisonings occuring in and around the home.

2. While the majority of calls (61%) represent events involving children under age 5, the precentage of reported ingestions in ages 0-5 has continually been dropping since 1972.

3. An increasing number of calls since 1972 involve adolescents and young adults (ages 12-24). These represent 14% of ingestions in 1974 vs. 9.7% of ingestions in 1972.

4. 1974 total calls increased by 45.9% over 1973's figure. In the same time period, there was 6.7% decrease in the 1974 vs. 1973 use of selected local Maryland emergency room visits for poisoning ingestions. Increased call rates may indicate increased awareness of MPIC services and/or a decrease in the use of other forms of post-injury care.

Expanding Media to Increase Public Awareness: The
Mr. Yuk Program

The impetus to expand MPIC mass media poison preven-
tion programs evolved from interests of a Metropolitan
Baltimore community organization, the Randallstown
Jaycees. Through combined efforts of the Jaycees and
the MPIC, funds enabling the MPIC to join the National
Poison Center Network were obtained from Blue Cross-
Blue Shield of Maryland, and the Mellon Foundation.

Motivation to join this network was influenced by the
availability of a poison prevention public education
program. This program provides television and radio
spot announcements, billboard materials and self-adhesive
poison warning labels to be affixed to hazardous substance containers. The television spots were prepared
for the Pittsburgh Poison Center by a professional film
making firm.

While the Pittsburgh program was developed in 1971
as a focus for a major state and regional public education poison prevention program, no formal evaluation
has been conducted on outcomes of this tool for information dissemination. The Pittsburgh Center intuitively
believes, however, that its program has made major impact on reported ingestions over several years.

The Pittsburgh program is known as the Mr. Yuk program
because of its innovative copyrighted warning symbol
(Figure 1). The idea for a new poison warning symbol
evolved from studies indicating that the traditional
warning symbol of skull and crossbones had lost its
effectiveness in Pittsburgh where children associated
this symbol with the Pittsburgh Pirates baseball team,
pirates in general, and a sense of excitement and ad-
venture. In a test program conducted at Pittsburgh
day care centers to develop a new warning symbol,
children were shown identical bottles of amber fluid
each with a unique warning symbol. Children were asked

to identify any bottle with which they would not play. The least attractive symbol for the children was a negative version of the familiar bright yellow, smiley-face button. The symbol was named Mr. Yuk by a child in the study group who declined to pick up the bottle marked with the green scowling face because "he looks yukky."

The Pittsburg study also found that many parents did not know whom to contact in the event their children ingested a suspected poisonous substance. Therefore, the name and emergency telephone number of the poison center were combined with the Mr. Yuk symbol in the form of a non-toxic sticker affixable on bottles and other containers housing dangerous substances such as medicines, cleaning fluids, etc. On request, at no cost, a sheet of twelve stickers is made available to the public. A donation is requested for additional sheets. A free brochure is mailed with the stickers identifying products on which they should be applied.

The Mr. Yuk program has three educational goals: (1) to encourage adults to affix a warning label on substance containers with potentially hazardous substances when ingested; (2) to encourage adults to inform their children that wherever the Mr. Yuk symbol appears it signifies danger, which means do not touch; and (3) to inform adults or younger childcare keepers of the PIC emergency telephone number for use in the event of substance ingestion. However, as noted above, the Mr. Yuk program has not been evaluated to measure the extent to which it meets these goals.

Evaluating Mr. Yuk's Effect in Maryland

I. Background: Throughout Metropolitan Baltimore, the MPIC in collaboration with the Randallstown Jaycees, undertook the implementation of the Mr. Yuk program. Mr. Yuk television spots were supplemented by other educational activities including public talks to

community groups; press releases to local newspapers;
and the distribution of Mr. Yuk stickers in public
access facilities, such as pharmacies, private doctor's
offices, clinics and hospital emergency rooms throughout
the area. In addition, a telephone survey was designed
to measure the effectiveness of these activities in
meeting one of the three educational goals of the Mr. Yuk
program: to inform the public of the PIC emergency
telephone number for use in the event of substance
ingestion.

The incentive to evaluate the Mr. Yuk program was also
based on a broader recognition that despite exorbitant
expenditures for public health information and educational efforts, little or no evaluation is conducted
to determine effectiveness of such actions in altering
personal or community health behavior. Studies conducted by the President's Committee on Health Education,
for example, reveal that while the five major voluntary
health agencies in the United States have annual expenditures amounting to $100 million for informational mate-
rial, there is relatively little concern in evaluating
whether the information got the message across. In contrast to these vast expenditures by voluntary agencies,
the President's Committee found that health education
is a highly underfinanced activity in government and
industry. In 1972, DHEW spent $30 million of its $18.2
billion budget for health education activities. In
addition $7 billion for health was allocated to other
federal agencies. However, except for the Department
of Defense, 26 other federal agencies did not know how
health education dollars were being spent (8).

We felt committed to determine the extent to which
our dollars in Maryland might effect poison ingestion
outcomes. The extent to which the Mr. Yuk program
succeeds in informing the public about MPIC may bear
on many findings about mass media and health-related
behavior. Young (9) in reviewing research related to
health education communication, shows that mass media

generally succeeds in reaching a majority of the public and stimulating the learning of at least partially correct information. Other studies show that while television is an effective advertising medium, its persuasive influence over purchasing habits may not extend equally to other matters such as health. In effect, while television does increase intensity or motivation, it rarely alters the nature of that motivation. Television appears to be most effective in directing ways in which a product or service will meet already known needs (10).

The potential of using mass media to advance the health of the nation was explored by health education specialists and experts from the entertainment industry at a special conference on health education in 1973 (11). To evaluate mass media for this purpose, an important distinction between health information vs. health educations was made; i.e., according to the findings and recommendation of the President's Committee on Health Education, health information refers to the production of materials (pamphlets, brochures, films, film strips, media use, etc.) while health education refers to methods which would help an individual act upon exposure to the printed or spoken word (12).

Because 95% of homes in the United States have at least one television and Americans view television on the average of six hours daily, one cannot deny the tremendous public exposure opportunity. The entertainment industry provides the following suggestions to the health industry to facilitate the use of television for health education purposes (13). The following summary of these suggestions are presented in terms of the extent to which they have been applied to the MPIC Mr. Yuk program:

1. Think of selling health as a product, like any other product would be sold. There are four television spots; a 60 and 30 second spot for

children. The <u>Mr. Yuk</u> children's spots are slick,
color-animated cartoons with catchy words and music.
The product for sale is <u>Mr. Yuk</u>, the symbol itself,
and it is very well packaged. The adult spots, on
the other hand, are more dramatic episodes, vi-
gnettes much like one views for the use of over-
the-counter medicines for the relief of nagging
backache. Anecdotally, many adult viewers are
more familiar with the children's <u>vs</u>. the adult's
spots.

2. <u>Think in terms of targeted communication strategy</u>.
As McLuhan points out, communication is a system
which includes the sender, the receiver, the
medium, the message and the response: what do
you want from the receiver? <u>Mr. Yuk</u> television
spots clearly send messages to the viewer (receiver)
of what response is desirable: "<u>Mr. Yuk</u> is mean,
<u>Mr. Yuk</u> is green," get this warning device, put
it on your hazardous products, call your local
poison center in event of emergency. The PIC
message, however, which conveys the emergency
phone number, has less impact than any other part
of the announcement. It appears on the screen
very quickly, for a short time, and the number is
not verbally announced. The words "poison information center" are used only once. Since many
television viewers <u>listen</u> to television without
<u>watching</u> it, it would be more effective if the
PIC phone number were announced and the poison
information center mentioned several times.

3. <u>Think in terms of using professional communicators</u>.
<u>Mr. Yuk</u> was created and designed by a commercial
professional communications firm for the Pittsburgh
Poison Center.

4. <u>Program to reach audience with effective prime
time</u>. The four spots announcements are shown
at varying times of day and night on four

commercial Maryland television stations. The
MPIC has no control over time of day or frequency
of showings. However, no concerted educational
attempts, persuasive measures or other incentives
were conveyed to the local television stations in
attempt to alter their program plans.

5. Increase efforts to enlist people the public
admires. Mr. Yuk utilizes this principle by
attempting to create Mr. Yuk as a public hero
who warns of impending doom, particularly for
children who consume products bearing his symbol.

6. Seek support from America's business corporation.
In addition to University funding, financial support enabling the MPIC to join the National Poison
Information Network, and to use the Mr. Yuk program, was contributed by Blue Cross-Blue Shield
of Maryland and the Mellon Foundation.

II. Evaluation Methods: In February 1975, prior to
the onset of the Mr. Yuk program, a baseline measure
was established through a random sample telephone survey
in Metropolitan Baltimore to determine emergency service
systems known and used by laypeople in post-injury periods. After 8 months, a second random sample of similar size in the same area was surveyed by phone. Two
hundred calls were completed in both pre and post-tests.
Telephone numbers for both the pre and post-tests were
selected randomly through the combined use of the
Metropolitan Baltimore phone directory, a random numbers
generator and a random numbers table. All non-residential
phone numbers were excluded.

Structured pre and post interview forms were designed.
Two MPIC employees conducted pre-test calls (Table I);
one employee completed the post-test (Table II). Calls
were made sequentially from the prepared numbers list.
If the phone was busy, disconnected, or there was no
answer the caller proceeded to the next number on the

list. If someone answered the phone, the interviewer asked: "Is this - " and repeated the dialed number. If the response indicated an incorrectly dialed number, the call was terminated and the correct number dialed. If the response was "yes," the interviewer said:

"I am calling from the University of Maryland. We are conducting a telephone survey and would appreciate your answering a few questions. (Pause) If you or one of your family members used or swallowed a commercial product or a drug in a manner that you thought was harmful, what would you do?"

The response was recorded verbatim on the interview sheet (Table I).

The questionnaire sought the following information about the PIC:

1. Whether the respondent would name the PIC as a resource in the event of a potentially hazardous ingestion; and if so,

2. Whether the respondent said he/she knew the PIC phone number; and if not,

3. Whether the respondent knew how to get the PIC phone number.

In the pre-test, data were also obtained to estimate costs for direct service emergency care used in the event of poison ingestions. Cost estimates are based on Blue Cross-Blue Shield of Maryland emergency coverage. Because Blue Cross-Blue Shield coverage includes ambulance and emergency room use, when a respondent indicated that an ambulance would be called or that the victim would be taken to a hospital or emergency room, the respondent was asked whether he/she had health insurance; and if so, whether it was Blue

Cross-Blue Shield.*

The post-test (Table II) was used to determine if the Mr. Yuk program led to changes in action following the possible ingestion of a commercial product or drug that was considered harmful. In the post-test the respondent was asked if he/she had "ever heard the name Mr. Yuk." If yes, the person was asked "Who is Mr. Yuk and how did you hear of him?" This information was recorded verbatim. If the respondent had not heard of Mr. Yuk, the interviewer read the following statement:

"Mr. Yuk is a new poison warning symbol that is designed to replace the skull and crossbones and to warn young children of a poisoning danger."

Post-test subjects were also asked if they had ever heard or seen a commercial about the Maryland Poison Information Center. They were also asked if they would like to be sent information about the MPIC prevention poison and emergency care. If yes, the respondent was asked for a mailing address; and materials were then disseminated. The call was terminated by thanking the respondent for participating.

III. Results: To complete 200 calls to both the pre and post-tests, 292 phone numbers were called in the pre-test and 387 in the post-test. Table III explains why the extra calls were needed and demonstrates a very low refusal rate in both tests.

Table IV presents information on where respondents seek help for poison ingestions. In the pre-test, 61.5%, and in the post-test 46% of the respondents said they would first turn to traditional health care

---

*Cost estimates are restricted here to Blue Cross-Blue Shield insurees. Blue Cross-Blue Shield provided partial funding to undertake the Mr. Yuk program.

providers, local physicians and hospital emergency rooms when faced with a potential poisoning emergency. In both pre and post-test, between one-fifth and one-fourth, said they would use a home remedy as the total treatment or as a first treatment procedure before contacting a direct service or information facility.

In the pre-test, 24 of 200 respondents said they would seek help from the MPIC: this number increased by five in the post-test. When we examine how easily pre and post-test groups would be able to reach the MPIC, we find that one-third in the pre-test (7 of 24) and half in the post-test (14 of 29) knew the MPIC phone number, had it listed in their personal phone directory, or had a label with the number affixed to the telephone (Table V). While this does not represent a statistically significant increase at .05 level, it is significant at the .16 level. We may then assume the probability that 84% of the time the observed shift in pre-post test periods did not occur by chance. However, we cannot attribute this shift to the Mr. Yuk program, the major organized public activity for disseminating information about the MPIC during the study period.

Table VI presents post-test results of exposure to any of the four Mr. Yuk television spots. 57.8% (115 of 199)* said that they had heard or seen one of the television spots. Since our objective was to increase awareness about the Poison Center as well as to introduce Mr. Yuk, our assumption was that those people who had heard of Mr. Yuk would be the same group that had seen the MPIC spot. This in fact was not the case as Table VI demonstrates. As the row totals indicate, 62% (75) of the 121 people who had heard of Mr. Yuk said that they had seen a commercial about the MPIC. However, of the 78 people who had not heard of Mr. Yuk, 51.3% (40) said that they had heard or seen a television spot about MPIC. Since the spots emphasize Mr. Yuk with more fervor than MPIC, this appears as an interesting observation. We are unable to discern specifically how these individuals heard about the MPIC. Possible intervening

variables are the telephone directory, written flyers
through personal contact with someone exposed to the
media or the center itself.

Summary and Implications

A pre and post phone survey to evaluate the success
of a large Metropolitan PIC through the use of media
reveals:

1. 19.1% of respondents in post vs. pre test were
    more knowledgeable about the presence of the
    MPIC and how to reach it in post-injury periods.

2. 121 or 200 post-test respondents knew the name
    Mr. Yuk, the new symbol for poison prevention;
    75% of these people also heard about MPIC.

3. Over an eight month period, 40,000 sheets of
    Mr. Yuk stickers were mailed on request to
    Metropolitan Baltimore residents.

There are two major forces which we believe limit
Mr. Yuk's power to motivate viewers into action intended
by his message.

1. Economics: Differences between health education
    messages and commercial announcements are that
    the latter are selectively projected at consid-
    erable costs to reach specific target populations
    at specific prime times; health education mes-
    sages on the other hand depend on random pro-
    gram content, special news reports and charit-
    able public service announcements. Although
    the networks are required by the FCC to run a
    certain number of spots/month, many are seen
    between 2:00 and 6:00 a.m. These placed defi-
    nite constraints on the Mr. Yuk television
    spots, whose scheduling is at the discretion of

station programmers. Stations can give us, as
researchers, no accounting about time and frequency of exposure over the eight months of our
study.

2. Psychology: Owing to economic constraints and
   public viewing habits, only a certain percentage
   of the population will be exposed to health information or education. As Swinehart of the
   Children's Television Network notes (16):

   "Many peoply are not exposed to the messages,
   some who see them pay little attention, some
   who learn do not accept the messages, some
   who accept them are not motivated to act,
   some who are motivated to act fail to do so."

We know that over an eight month period, 40,000
sheets of Mr. Yuk stickers were mailed on request to
residents of Metropolitan Baltimore.

However, since the optimum measure of disseminating
public health education is overt behavior corresponding
to the health message, a second activity to evaluate
public reaction to the Mr. Yuk program would be justi-
fied. Survey data would be useful in identifying
demographic characteristics in a population sample
requesting Mr. Yuk stickers, how these stickers are
used and where household products and medicines are
stored. Also valuable, would be a comparison between
poison ingestions reported by households using and
not using Mr. Yuk stickers.

REFERENCES

1. Fonaroff A, Hodes B: Injurious effects of the drug use process: An analysis of ingested non-prescribed drug products reported to a poison information center. *Drugs in Health Care* 3:35-49, 1976.

2. Fonaroff A: The community as an environmental system in which accidents occur. *American Public Health Association Annual Meeting, Injury Control Section*, November 1974.

3. Verhulst HL, Crotty JJ: Childhood poison accidents. *JAMA* 203:12:145-146, 1968.

4. Crotty JJ: Personal communication to the author, November 10, 1975.

5. Bureau of Product Safety, Poison Control. *National Child Health and Development Statistics, p 10*. Washington, DC, 1972-1973.

6. Maryland Poison Information Center: *Annual Statistical Report - 1974*. University of Maryland School of Pharmacy.

7. Maryland Poison Information Center: *Annual Statistical Report - 1974*. University of Maryland School of Pharmacy.

8. Weingarten V: Report of findings and recommendations of the President's committee on health education, in Reader G (ed): *Health Education Monograph 2, Suppl 1*. 1974.

9. Young MAC: Review of research and studies related to health education communication: Methods and materials. *Health Education Monographs* 25:55-57, 1967.

10. Young MAC: Review of research and studies

related to health education communication: Methods and materials. *Health Education Monographs* 25:55-57, 1967.

11. Reader G (ed): *Proceedings of the Will Rogers Conference on Health Education, Monograph 2, Suppl 1,* 1974.

12. Weingarten V: Report of finding and recommendations of the President's committee on health education, in Reader G (ed): *Health Education Monograph 2,* 1974.

13. Siebert WA: Health education and television communication, in Reader (ed): *Proceedings of the Will Rogers Conference on Health Education,* monograph 2, 1973.

14. Maryland Poison Information Center: *Annual Statistical Report - 1974.* University of Maryland School of Pharmacy.

15. Moriarity R: Personal communication, 1974; and Veltri J: personal communication, 1975.

16. Swinehart JW: Comment on Thornton's paper, in *Health Education Monograph 2* 3:210, 1974.

TABLE I

MPIC PRE-MEDIA PHONE SURVEY

INTERVIEW SHEET

DIRECTIONS:

1. Complete each question before moving to the next.
2. Ask each question exactly as it is worded here.
3. Record answers verbatim.

Phone Number _____

Hello - Is this _____? I am calling from the University of Maryland. We'r
                 phone number
conducting a telephone survey and would appreciate your answering a few questions:

1. If you or one of your family members used or swallowed a commercial product
   or a drug in a manner that you thought was harmful, what would you do?
   (Record verbatim).

If the person answers "call a Poison Center," ask questions listed under number 2.

If the person suggests taking him/her in a hospital, calling a hospital or calling an
ambulance, go to question 3.

For all other responses proceed to number 4.

                    (TO BE ANSWERED ONLY IF RESPONSE TO 1 IS POISON CENTER)

2. (a) Do you know the number of the Poison Center?   _____   _____
                                                             yes   no

   (b) If no, how would you obtain the phone number?

                    (TO BE ANSWERED ONLY IF RESPONSE TO 1 WAS HOSPITAL OR AMBULANCE)

3. (a) Do you have health insurance to help cover the expense?

            _____ _____ _____
              yes   no   don't know
   (b) If yes, what kind of insurance is it, or which company?

4. Thank you for your help.

        Your Name _____

TABLE II

MPIC FOLLOW-UP PHONE SURVEY

INTERVIEW SHEET

DIRECTIONS:

1. Complete each question before moving on to the next.
2. Ask each question exactly as it is worded here.
3. Record answers verbatim.

Phone Number _____

Hello - Is this _____? I am calling from the University of Maryland. We're
                phone number
conducting a telephone survey and would appreciate your answering a few questions:

1. If you or one of your family members used or swallowed a commercial product
   or a drug in a manner that you thought was harmful, what would you do?
   (Record verbatim). _____

   _____

IF THE PERSON ANSWERS "CALL THE POISON CENTER" ASK QUESTIONS LISTED UNDER QUESTION 2.
   FOR ALL OTHER RESPONSES PROCEED TO QUESTION 3).

2. (a) Do you know the number of the Poison Center?

        _____   _____   (IF NO, ASK B)
         yes   no

   (b) (IF NO) How would you obtain the phone number?

3. Have you ever heard the name Mr. Yuk? ___(IF YES GO TO A) ___(IF NO, GO TO B)
                                             yes   no

   (a) Who is Mr. Yuk and how did you hear of him? (Record verbatim). _____

   _____

                    (IF NO READ THE FOLLOWING STATEMENT)

   (b) Mr. Yuk is a new poison warning symbol that is designed to replace the skull
        and crossbones and to warn young children of a poisoning danger.

4. Have you ever heard a commercial about the Maryland Poison Information Center?

        _____   _____
         yes   no

5. Would you like me to send you some information about the Poison Center?

        _____   _____   (IF YES PROCEED WITH THE FOLLOWING QUESTION)
         yes   no

IF YES ASK: "MAY I HAVE YOUR ADDRESS AND ZIP CODE." RECORD DIRECTLY ON ENVELOPE. IF
THE PERSON DOES NOT GIVE HIS NAME

(IF YES ASK: "MAY I HAVE YOUR ADDRESS AND ZIP CODE." RECORD DIRECTLY ON ENVELOP. IF
THE PERSON DOES NOT GIVE HIS NAME, ADDRESS ENVELOPE TO RESIDENT. DO NOT ASK FOR NAME.)

6. Thank you very much for your help.

    YOUR NAME_____ DATE_____

TABLE III

OUTCOMES OF MPIC TELEPHONE CALLS IN PRE/POST TEST PERIODS

	Pre Test	Post Test
reed to Participate	200	200
fused to Participate	17	27
Answer	44	89
ɔne Disconnected	28	60
ɜy Signal	3	7
Adult Present	0	4
TOTALS	292	387

Table IV

Where People Seek Help for Poison Ingestions*

	Pre Test		Post Test	
	#	%	#	%
Call or Take to Doctor	69	34.5	59	29.5
Call or Take to Hospital	54	27.0	33	16.5
Home Remedy	41	20.5	48	24.0
POISON CENTER	24	12.0	29	14.5
Ambulance	5	2.5	9	4.5
From Label on Ingested Item	4	2.0	5	2.5
Call Pharmacist	1	0.5	0	0
Call Police	0	0	2	1.0
Don't Know	2	1.0	11	5.5
Other	0	0	4	2.0
TOTALS	200	100	200	100

*In some cases, the respondent's answer contained more than one action.
For example, the first response might not be to seek information but to
proceed directly with a home remedy, such as one producing emesis. This
act might then be followed by calling the MPIC, a doctor, or taking the
ingestor to a hospital. Results in Table IV do not show multiple responses
the table presents data only for the first response given since there
was not a significant difference between the response and other remarks
made.

TABLE V

OW PEOPLE SAY THEY WOULD OBTAIN THE POISON CENTER PHONE NUMBER

	Pre Test		Post Test	
	#	%	#	%
all Operator	9	37.5	2	6.9
new Phone Number (Had it listed in personal phone directory or had telephone sticker on telephone with MPIC number)	7	29.2	14	48.3
one Book	7	29.2	10	34.5
re Department	1	4.2	0	0
t Listed	0	0	2	6.9
her	0	0	1	3.4
TOTALS	24	100.1	29	100.0

TABLE VI

NUMBER OF PEOPLE WHO DID AND DID NOT SEE A

MR. YUK TELEVISION SPOT

	Number of People Who Heard or Saw Television Spot about MPIC	Number of People Who Did Not Hear of See Television Spot about MPIC	TOTALS
Number Heard of Mr. Yuk	75	46	121 Heard of Mr. Yuk
Number did Not Hear of Mr. Yuk	40	38	78 Never Heard of Mr. Yuk
	115 Who Heard or Saw Television Spot	84 Who Never Heard or Saw Television Spot	

----

*The 200th respondent did not know whether he/she had seen television spot.

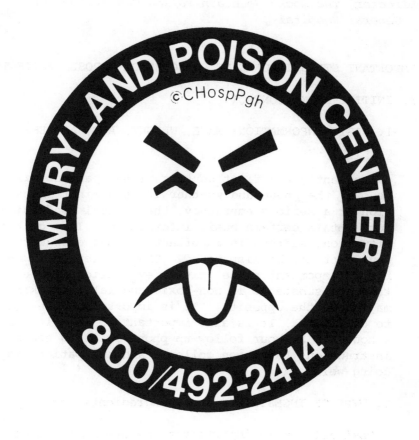

Figure 1. The MPIC <u>Mr. Yuk</u> Warning Symbol

MANAGEMENT OF ACUTE POISONING AND OVERDOSE

Barry H. Rumack, M.D.
*The Departments of Pediatrics and Medicine and the
Division of Clinical Pharmacology
The University of Colorado Medical Center
Director, The Rocky Mountain Poison Center, Denver
General Hospital*

IMPORTANT STEPS IN CARE OF POISONED OR EXPOSED PATIENTS

A. INITIAL PHONE CONTACT

1. BASIC INFORMATION: NAME, WEIGHT, AGE, ADDRESS,
PHONE

Frequently the first contact with a patient will
be over the phone and whether it is a minor ingestion or a serious emergency, the medical profession
must obtain certain basic information. In a critical
situation, address is important so that emergency
equipment may be dispatched. Their telephone number is important since initial evaluation may be
that the substance is non-toxic and later checking
may prove the opposite. It is important to be able
to call back. It is also important to do a 1 hour,
4 hour and 24 hour follow-up phone call and see if
instructions have been followed and the patient is
doing well.

2. TYPE OF INGESTION - name, ingredients, amount

Obviously it is important to determine the type
of ingestion so that specific consideration for
treatment can be made. Caution must be observed
since approximately 50% of all histories at this
point are incorrect either as to agent, amount or
consumption.

3. EVALUATION OF SEVERITY

Is life in: Immediate Danger
            Potential Danger
            No Danger

This evaluation will determine whether or not the patient can be transported to the hospital by private means or by emergency vehicle and, indeed, if the patient actually needs to come to the hospital at all. If the decision is to bring the patient to the hospital, then:

HAVE THE POISON, THE CONTAINERS, AND EVERYTHING QUESTIONABLE IN THE AREA BROUGHT WITH THE PATIENT

4. DECONTAMINATION

SKIN - If the patient has been exposed to an acid, alkali, insecticide, gasoline, or anything else which can burn the skin or be absorbed, it is important to decontaminate the skin and avoid further toxicity. If the patient needs ventilatory assistance, is in shock, etc., then decontamination may not be possible until patient is stabilized. Use plain water or soap and water or green soap in copious amounts with soft non-abrasive sponge or cloth. Protect medical personnel.

INTERNAL - Unless the patient is comatose, seizing or has lost the gag reflex, it is always safe to give a few glasses of milk or water and dilute the material. Then syrup of ipecac, if appropriate, may be administered and the patient brought in.

5. ALERT THE EMERGENCY DEPARTMENT

Provide as many details as possible so that ED personnel will be ready with necessary equipment.

6. SAVE ALL EMESIS - If the patient vomits, collect and save all of it in a clean bowl and bring it to the hospital with the patient.

7. POISON PREVENTION - If the ingestion is clearly non-toxic and there are no symptoms, then it is useful to provide a short piece of poison prevention over the phone.

Poison Prevention Over the Phone

A few simple questions may reveal hazardous substances stored in unsafe locations. The following list will help discover various substances in key areas of a home:

    drain cleaning crystals liquid
    dishwasher soap and cleaning supplies
    paints and thinners
    medicines
    garden sprays and materials
    automobile products

If there are problems in the home, it will be useful to schedule the patient for a discussion or to dispatch a public health nurse. Multiple ingestors are sometimes a form of child battering and appropriate referral is critical. If a parent has become hysterical over a minor problem - such as sucking on a ballpoint pen - then it may be useful to have an immediate visit to calm the situation.

Prevention of Poisoning

A major goal of physicians is to reduce the number of accidental ingestions in the high risk age group under five years old. A systematic poison education effort should be part of the routine care of every patient. Awareness of

potential hazards and raising of consciousness
among parents has recently been made significantly
easier through the character known as "Officer Ugg"
(Fig. 1). Parents of very young children are encouraged to search the house and identify all
hazardous substances. As the child is gradually
taught the meaning of the face, then parents and
children can play "poison policeman" and together
identify hazardous substances. Children are taught
to imitate the face and cover their mouths whenever
confronted with a potential toxic situation, whether
or not the sticker face is attached. A Royalty
Free License for the use of this symbol as part of
any poison education program is available from the
Rocky Mountain Poison Foundation, 1722 Prudential
Plaza, Denver, Colorado 80202.

B. INITIAL EMERGENCY ROOM CONTACT

1. FIRST see if the patient is BREATHING

   This is sometimes overlooked in the emergency
   room frenzy of getting IV lines started and
   running to get the poison book, etc.

2. Check adequacy of the TIDAL VOLUME. Normal is
   10-15 cc/kg.

3. IS THE PATIENT IN SHOCK? If so, avoid pressors
   initially and administer fluids plasmanate or blood.

4. Skin decontamination - if it has not been done,
   it must now be done. If emergency personnel have
   come in contact with the material, they must also
   be decontaminated, especially, for example, if it
   is organophosphate which may be absorbed through
   the skin. Emergency Department personnel should
   wear disposable plastic gloves and aprons to protect themselves while decontaminating patients.

5. HISTORY - Additional or complete history should
be taken from family, friends, or patient if possible. This may have to be done by someone not on
the primary care team if the patient is quite ill.

NOW THAT EMERGENCY PROCEDURES HAVE BEEN PERFORMED,
EACH PATIENT MUST BE EVALUATED IN THREE AREAS:

1. Can further absorption be prevented:

   Skin decontamination
   Emesis
   Lavage
   Charcoal
   Cathartic

2. Can enhancement of exercises of the poison be
   be achieved?

   Forced diuresis
   Peritoneal dialysis
   Hemodialysis
   Exchange transfusion
   Hemoperfusion

3. Can symptoms be treated with specific physiologic
   antagonists?

   The remainder of this paper will deal with
   these three areas.

TREATMENT INFORMATION

   Books available to provide poison information
are in general several years out of date. Information contained on labels of products are similarly
out of date and may be incorrect. The POISINDEX
system is a computer generated microfiche emergency
poison management system which is kept up to date
at quarterly intervals. The entire system is re-

published every 3 months and in addition to treatment information contains the largest compendium in the world of product ingredient data. Colorfiche of plants, snakes and mushrooms are included as well as an alphabetical and a numerical listing of all drug imprint codes.

Clinical Evaluation

In addition to the usual physical examination, several scoring systems for coma, hyperactivity and withdrawal have been developed. They are useful not just to obtain the score but to remember to check certain key points. It is also very valuable to follow these and see if the patient is improving or deteriorating.

CLASSIFICATION OF COMA

0 Asleep, but can be aroused and can answer questions
1 Comatose, does withdraw from painful stimuli, reflexes intact
2 Comatose, does NOT withdraw from painful stimuli, most reflexes intact, no respiratory or circulatory depression
3 Comatose, most or all reflexes are absent but without depression of respiration or circulation
4 Comatose, reflexes absent, respiratory depression with cyanosis, circulatory failure or shock

CLASSIFICATION OF HYPERACTIVITY

1+ Restlessness, irritability, insomnia, tremor, hyperreflexia, sweating, mydriasis, flushing
2+ Confusion, hyperactivity, hypertension, tachypnea, tachycardia, extra systoles, sweating, mydriasis, flushing, mild hyperpyrexia

3+ Delirium, mania, self-injury, marked hypertension, tachycardia, arrhythmias, hyperpyrexia
4+ Above plus: convulsions, coma, circulatory
collapse

CLASSIFICATION OF WITHDRAWAL

Score the following findings on a 0,1,2 point basis

diarrhea	hypertension	restlessness
dilated pupils	insomnia	tachycardia
goose flesh	lacrimation	yawning
hyperactive bowel sounds	muscle cramps	

1-5 mild
6-10 moderate
11-15 severe

**Seizures indicate severe withdrawal regardless of
the rest of the score.**

TO VOMIT OR NOT TO VOMIT

It must now be decided whether or not emesis is
indicated. Specific CONTRAINDICATIONS to emesis are:

strong acids or bases
patient is unconscious, seizing, or lost the gag
reflex
hydrocarbons (this is very controversial-see the
great hydrocarbon debate on page 9)[*]

If none of these conditions exist, induced emesis
should be used even if it has been several hours
since ingestion. Many drugs delay gastric emptying
time and some like salicylates may form a mass in
the stomach which may remain for several days slowly
releasing its toxic substance. Emesis should be

done NO MATTER what the time lag was until arrival at your facility.

How to Vomit

1. Ipecac - The most readily available drug for induction of vomiting is syrup of ipecac (not the elixer or fluid extract, which is toxic). It is inexpensive ($0.50 - 1.00), keeps well, can be administered at home, and by law may be dispensed in 30 cc aliquots without prescription. It should be routinely given to mothers with small children at the baby's 6 month or 1 year check-up along with a prevention discussion.

Give a child 1 tablespoon (15 cc) of Syrup of Ipecac with 1-2 glasses of water or Kool Aid and activity.

Adult dose 30 cc (2 tablespoons)
Pediatric dose 15 cc (1/2 oz., 1 tblsp.) orally,
            repeated 1 time if necessary

Method   a) give ipecac orally
         b) follow with large amounts of whatever
            fluid the child will drink (ipecac on
            an empty stomach is like squeezing an
            empty balloon)
         c) keep the patient ambulatory
         d) after 15 minutes stimulate the patient's
            throat to help emesis
         e) should work in 20-30 minutes - suspect
            tranquilizer (antiemetic) if doesn't

2. Apomorphine - This will readily induce vomiting but has several problems: it does not keep well on the shelf in liquid form, it cannot be administered at home, it is not readily available, and it may cause respiratory depression which outlasts the reversant. It is not advised in children.

Dose   0.1 mg/kg IV or sub-Q
CAUTION Do not use apomorphine unless a
reversing agent is available (See below)

Method a) Usually a 6 mg tablet in an unsterile
container is available. Add 3 cc of
diluent for a final concentration of
2 mg/cc.
b) If the patient is in critical need to
vomit immediately, this preparation
can be given IV. If the patient does
not need emesis immediately, give the
dose sub-Q.
c) give large quantities of oral fluids
d) emesis should ensue in 5-15 minutes
e) do not repeat the dose

Reversal of Apomorphine. Naloxone (Narcan)
0.005 mg/kg should be given as soon as adequate
emesis has been obtained. Usual adult dose 0.4
mg IV; usual pediatric dose 0.1 mg IV. Nalorphine
(Nalline) 0.1 mg/kg may be used if Naloxone is unavailable.

3. Other Emetics. Sodium chloride is very dangerous.
Fatalities due to hypernatremia have been reported.
Mustard powder is questionably effective. There must
be 10 or more other things proposed, all of which are
at best questionably effective.

4. Save all Emesis. The initial emesis should be
put in a urine or stool container and saved separately
from the rest of the emesis. All emesis produced
should be saved and sent to the laboratory.

* The great hydrocarbon debate - Most texts dealing
with hydrocarbons as an absolute contraindication to
emesis. Instead "cautious gastric lavage" is stated
as therapy of choice. Cautious gastric lavage in an
awake child does not exist. There is now evidence to
show that aspiration pneumonia is twice as common follow-

ing lavage for hydrocarbons than it is following ipecac emesis. The following is a reasonable approach to hydrocarbon ingestion.

1. If the patient has taken 1 cc/kg of hydrocarbon or less of a chlorinated or metal containing solvent, CNS or respiratory depression may occur. If depression has occurred do not vomit, intubate with a cuffed endotracheal tube and perform gastric lavage, administer a cathartic and provide other supportive measures.

2. If the patient has taken a possible toxic amount and has a good gag reflex, no CNS depression and is breathing normally, ipecac induced emesis should be used. The time to remove a potentially lethal amount of material from the stomach is before CNS, respiratory, or cardiac depression.

3. If the patient has clearly had less than 1/2cc/kg amount of non-chlorinated or non-metal containing hydrocarbon, then catharsis with magnesium or sodium sulfate should be adequate.

4. Mineral oil or other oil based cathartics should not be used since there is an increased risk of lipoid pneumonia. It has been clearly demonstrated that oils previously used to "thicken" ingested hydrocarbons do not work and provide some risk.

5. In any event, if there is any question as to aspiration, a chest x-ray should be taken. It used to be thought that aspiration pneumonia occurred as a result of emesis because initial x-rays showed a clear chest and after emesis a pneumonia. It is now obvious that this is not true and most aspirations occurs on the way down, not up. X-ray should be done at 1st sign of aspiration and if negative should be repeated if the patient is symptomatic at 6-8 hours.

6. If the patient arrives coughing, then aspiration is almost a certainty to have occurred but may not be evident on chest x-ray for 6-8 hours.

7. Steroids provide no assistance in treatment of of aspiration and may cause harm.

8. Epinephrine is CONTRAINDICATED as it may produce ventricular arrhythmias.

9. Antibiotics provide no prophylactic benefit and should not be used unless infection is documented.

THE OROGASTRIC HOSE

If a patient is becoming unconscious, is unconscious, has lost the gag reflex, or is seizing, endotracheal or nasotracheal intubation (the latter is preferred) followed by a large orogastric tube is the method of choice rather than vomiting. A 28 French Ewald is the SMALLEST that should be used and preferably a 36 Fr Ewald which is about 1 cm in diameter with large holes should be used. Some of the major European poison centers use this method almost exclusively for all ingestions. The usual size NG tube of 16 or 18 Fr is completely worthless except for liquids. Tablets cannot be aspirated through it. The preferred lavage solution is saline which should be warm after the 2nd liter to avoid lowering the patient's temperature. The patient should be in the left side head down position. Lavage should continue until no solid material returns. Rarely will all of the toxin be removed at this end point and other measures to prevent further absorption must be taken. If the ingestant is absorbed by charcoal,put charcoal in the lavage after obtaining the initial aspirate for analysis.

The large tubes have at least a 25 cc dead space to fill so that lavage should be no less than 50 cc. In an adult 300 cc is ideal perwash and in children

10 cc/kg wash is best. Do not exceed these maximums or there is a risk of washing through the pylorus.

LABORATORY

Specific laboratory tests and screens are available for compounds and groups of compounds. It is critical to consult the analytical chemist early so that correct samples can be obtained for the suspended poison. Discussing symptomatology and suspicions from history will help the analyst reach an answer more quickly. Sending specimens with a request for "poison screen" will take the analysis many hours and prolong identification so that definitive care can be delayed.

Supportive care should be provided while laboratory results are pending.

Specimens

1. Gastric contents

   a) emesis - save all emesis produced and send entire amount to laboratory so that qualitative determinations can be made.

   b) gastric lavage - save the initial aspirate separately from the large amount of lavage solution but send both to the laboratory.

2. Blood

   Discuss sample containers and amounts of blood with the analyst but in general, 10 cc of heparinized blood will usually suffice.

3. Urine

   100 cc of urine should be collected and sent

to the laboratory. In pediatric patients
less may be available.

Results

Positive identification of a drug is all that is
usually necessary. Drug levels are helpful in determining prognosis and in considering procedures
such as dialysis. Since patients fall on a normal
distribution of response, lack of clinical correlation with blood level may occur. Glutethimide levels,
for example, may be higher when the patient awakens
than when the patient came in with coma. Caution
must be exercised in interpretation of laboratory
test. For example, a salicylamide run as a standard
salicylate by Trinders technique will give a negative
result and may be missed. It must be done fluoromet-
rically. If Deferoxamine is given before an iron
sample is taken, the analyst must know this to interpret his results. Lomotil, for example, is not
detectable at this time by any laboratory method.

CHARCOAL AND CATHARTICS

The following list of drugs is well absorbed by
activated charcoal. It is important to remember that
activated charcoal is different than universal antidote which is burnt toast, magnesium oxide, and tannic
acid. It is much less effective than activated charcoal and tannic acid is potentially hepatotoxic.
Universal antidote has no place in Toxicology.

alcohol	cocaine	muscarine	phosphorous
amphetamines	digitalis	nicotine	potassium
antimony	glutethimide	opium	permangena
antipyrene	iodine	oxalates	quinine
atropine	IPECAC	parathion	salicylates
arsenic	malathion	penicillin	selenium
barbiturates	mercuric chloride	phenol	silver
camphor	methylene blue	phenolphthalein	stramonium
cantharides	morphine	phenothiazine	strychnine
			sulfonamide

Contraindications

There are no known contraindications to administration of charcoal. Since it adsorbs and inactivates
ipecac it is best to administer charcoal _after_ emesis.
If the ingestant is adsorbed by charcoal, put charcoal
down orally and then lavage. After emesis or lavage
give more charcoal. Since charcoal is an inert and
non-toxic substance to the human subject, there should
be no hesitation to use it if there is any doubt as to
when ingestion occurred. Some concern has been expressed about the occasional patient aspirating some
charcoal - no known adverse effects have occurred.

Dose and Method

The dose is 5 to 10 times the estimated weight of
the drug or chemical ingested. Usually 15-30 grams
in a slurry with water. If available for immediate
use, the charcoal-sorbital mixture can be used. It
is sweet and well tolerated. Don't delay until it
is made up, however.

Charcoal will also act as a marker of intestinal
transit time so that when it appears in the stool it
will be unlikely that any more absorption of drug
from the GI tract will occur.

Save All Gastric Material

The initial aspirate should be placed in a separate container. It will have the most concentrated
drug and laboratory identification will be easier.
Save all additional aspirate separately so that an
estimate of total drug aspirated can be made. Once
charcoal has been administered the aspirate may not
be of value to the laboratory.

CATHARTICS

Another useful mechanism to decrease potential drug toxicity is to move it rapidly through the GI tract so that absorption will be decreased.

Contraindications

Magnesium containing cathartics in renal failure. Oil based cathartics in pesticide poisoning.

As long as oil based cathartics are avoided, there are no contraindications to catharsis. Pneumonitis from aspiration of some of the oil based cathartics is a serious complication. Mineral oil pneumonia has been especially reported in this setting and is very difficult to treat. Even when large amounts of magnesium sulfate have given (100 gm over several hours) only insignificant rises will occur in serum magnesium.

Dose and Method

1. Magnesium sulfate (Epsom salts) with adult dose of 5 grams (or 50 cc of the 10% solution) and pediatric dosage of 250 mg/kg. 1 tablespoon (5 gram) mixed with honey or sweet liquid should produce effect in 2-4 hours. Repeat @ 2-4 hours until catharsis with charcoal in stool.

2. Fleets phospho-soda 15 to 30 ml diluted 1:4 of the material as it comes in the prepared bottles.

3. Sodium sulfate 250 mg/kg diluted 1:2 or 1:4.

4. ALL OF THESE AGENTS GIVEN ORALLY.

ANALEPTICS

Contraindicated

Doxapram, ethamivan, phenylmetertrazol, ritalin,

coramine, picrotoxin amphetamines and all others have
NO place in the treatment of the poisoned patient.
They clearly increase rather than decrease mortality
rates. A comatose patient receiving analeptics may
well turn into a seizing comatose patient. Don't
use them!

SURFACE DECONTAMINATION

Skin decontamination is essential following exposure
to substances that penetrate or burn the skin (caustics,
alkalies, acids, hydrocarbons, pesticides, cyanides).
The use of tincture of green soap is recommended since
bydrocarbons are more soluble in alcohol and it is alkaline which will hydrolyze the organophosphates.
Plain soap is useful, however, if green soap is not
readily available. It is important to clean thoroughly
the hair, umbilical area and under fingernails, toenails,
ears and groin but do not abrade the skin as it increases
the absorption of some chemicals. The person decontaminating a pesticide should take precautions not to get the
material on themselves. The patient's clothes and all
sheets, etc., that come in contact should be placed in
a plastic bag and marked. The use of substances that
will "neutralize" agents is not warranted. The use of
vinegar and lemon juice for all alkali materials, for
example, will create an exothermic reaction and burn
the patient. The use of emollients, such as greases
or oils, will simply make decontamination more difficult. The person decontaminating should wear disposable
gloves, apron and shoe covers.

EYE EXPOSURES

A young child may be wrapped in a sheet as a restraint.
Just pour irrigant on the eye as child will usually open
and close eyes making it unnecessary to pry the eye open.
Low pressure shower may be used for adult if immediately
available.

Irrigation of the EYE is the most important aspect
of the treatment and must be begun immediately. Initial
irrigation should occur at home with plain tap water.
Permanent irreversible destruction of the cornea can
occur in the 20 minutes it takes to come to the hospital. Tell them to irrigate for 20 minutes (by the
clock). Irrigation means holding the head back over
the sink and pouring saline or plain water from a
large pitcher or liter bottle into the affected eye.
Hold pitcher 6-8 inches from eye. The use of an eye-
dropper or irrigating syringe is worthless. The whole
idea behind irrigation is to dilute and remove the
agent quickly. It is best to have the first person
who sees the patient perform the irrigation rather
than delegate it to a nurse or aide who may not under-
stand the urgency and method. Irrigation should continue for 20 minutes with alkali and 5 minutes with
acid. All unknowns should, of course, be irrigated
for 20 minutes. Consultation with an ophthalmologist
is imperative. At minimum a steroid eye ointment
should be placed in the eye and patched.

ANTIDOTES - NECESSARY VERY EARLY IN COURSE

There are very few poisons that have a specific
antidote. The first 4 are the only ones that MUST be
administered immediately, as soon as there is suspicion
of the diagnosis. Often "antidotes" can be administered
after confirmation of the ingestion. Antidote implies
a substance that will reverse a poisoning by itself.
This is a risky concept as good supportive care MUST
be performed whether or not there is an antidote.

1. Carbon Monixide - oxygen

2. Cyanide - There should be a cyanide kit in every
   emergency room. The kit should have specific
   clear instructions as to the order of administration of amyl nitrite, sodium nitrite and sodium
   thiosulfate. The instructions and kit are de-

signed for adult emergencies and the instructions should be followed to the letter. The materials are packed in the order they should be used. Pharmacy must check drugs in kit yearly for expiration.

Adult Dose: Follow instructions in the kit.

Pediatric Dose: CAUTION: If the adult dose of sodium nitrate is given to a small child, potentially fatal methemoglobinemia may result. The dose of $NaNO_2$ for children with an average hemoglobin of 12 gm/100 ml is 10 mg/kg STAT and 5 mg/kg repeated within 30 minutes if necessary.

3. Nitrites and Nitrates - this also applies to aniline dyes and other methemoglobinemia producing toxins - methylene blue at 0.2 ml/kg IV over 5 minutes of a 1% solution in water. As a presumptive test for methemoglobinemia in a non-oxygen-responsive cyanotic patient, place 1 drop of your blood and 1 drop of the patient's blood on a filter paper. If the patient's blood is more chocolate than yours, then the patient probably has greater than 15% methemoglobinemia.

4. Organophosphate Insecticides - such as parathion and malathion - give atropine and 2-PAM. If an adult patient has small pupils and the odor of insecticides, then slowly give 2 mg atropine and observe. If the patient gets atropine effects gets and they cause problems, they can be reversed with physostigmine. Otherwise, continued doses of atropine will be necessary. The organophosphates are inhibitors of cholinesterase and atropine is a physiological antidote. The dose for children should be 0.05 mg/kg/initial dose. Start with atropine NOT 2-PAM. The dose of atropine may approach as much as 2 grams over a day. Be prepared to intubate.

OTHER ANTIDOTES

Long lists of "antidotes" appear in some articles.
These are usually treatments rather than true antidotes.
Other Clinical Toxicology lecture sheets are available
for specific treatments.

1. Amphetamines - chlorpromazine will help hyper-
   excitability 0.5 - 1.0 mg/kg IM.

2. Belladonna Alkaloids - physostigmine. Dose page 30.

3. Benadryl, Atropine, Potato Leaves, Asthmador,
   Jimsonweed - physostigmine. Dose page 30.

4. Heavy Metals - Specific chelation should be performed but the procedure should not be taken
   lightly. EDTA has significant toxicity, as do
   the other chelators, and the diagnosis should
   usually be confirmed before chelation therapy is
   begun.

5. Narcotics - Narcotic overdose, either with street
   drugs, Lomotil, Darvon, Talwin, or Methadone,
   occurs in non-addicts as well as addicts. In non-
   addicts respiratory care is more important than
   a specific antagonist. These patients can survive
   without an antagonist but with good respiratory
   care. Antagonists act very rapidly and should be
   used when available. They may not last as long
   as the depressant effects of the narcotic so that
   repeated doses may be necessary every 30-60 minutes. As many as 24 doses of Narcan have been
   used even if the patient is a suspected narcotic
   addict. Previous concern that patients would go
   into irreversible withdrawal has not been borne
   out and naloxone is clearly the drug of choice.
   It does not synergize or cause respiratory depression itself so can safely be used in any patient

Dose Naloxone (Narcan) 5-10 mcg (0.010 to 0.005 mg)/ kg/dose IV. Comes in 014 mg vials which is the usual adult dose. No respiratory depression occurs with use.

Nallorphine (Nalline) 01.mg/kg/dose. This is a second line drug which should be used only if naloxone is not available. It can cause significant respiration depression on its own.

6. Phenothiazines - Benadryl (2.5-5.0 mg/kg orally) is the first drug of choice for extrapyramidal findings, and may be necessary for a week to prevent return of symptoms.

7. Tricyclic Antidepressants - physostigmine. Use if there is arrhythmia or other difficulty with pulse or blood pressure. This is short acting and may have to be repeated. Alkalinization of the patient with bicarb has also been reported to give help in management.

FORCED DIURESIS

Forced diuresis is frequently useful in serious poisonings if the drug is excreted in the urine in active form. The technique should not be used unless it is specifically indicated, as it may increase the likelihood of cerebral edema, a common cause of death in the poisoned patient.

Some Drugs Helped by Forced Diuresis

alcohol
amphetamines (need acid diuresis)
bromides
isoniazid (usually big anion gaps, alkalinization needs will be massive)
other renally cleared drugs
phenobarbital (alkaline)
salicylates (need alkaline diuresis)
strychnine (acid)

Alkaline Diuresis can usually be accomplished with
bicarbonates, 1-2 mEq/kg IV. It is well to observe
for potassium depletion and administration of potassium citrate which has both potassium and considerable alkalizing ability may be used. It is also
available orally as K-Lyte "fizzies" which is a
quite palatable form. Follow serum K^+ loss.

Acid Diuresis may be accomplished with ascorbic acid,
arginine or ammonium chloride, all IV or orally.

1. Ascorbic acid may be given in doses of 500 mg
   to 2 gm orally or intravenously as needed to
   obtain acid urine (pH between 4.5 to 5.5).

2. Ammonium chloride may be used at a total dose
   of 2-6 gm/day or 75 mg/kg/dose in four divided
   doses. It comes as IV solution, tablets or syrup.

3. Many times Mannital diuresis will accomplish
   an acid urine alone without any additional
   measures.

Diuresis - Hypertonic or pharmacologic diuretics
should be given along with adequate fluids. Usual
urine flow is 0.5-2 ml/kg/hour and with forced diuresis
should be 3-6 ml/kg/hour. Alkaline or acid diuresis
should be chosen on the basis of the drug's PK_a so
that ionized drug will be trapped in the tubular
lumen and not reabsorbed. Osmotic load is also important and either type of diuretic should be given
at intervals. Reabsorption proximally will occur if
inadequate osmotic load is not maintained in the
tubule.

DIALYSIS

Hemodialysis (or peritoneal dialysis if hemodialysis
is unavailable) is useful in the poisonings detailed
below. It should be reserved for those patients in the

immediate category or those patients fitting the following criteria. Dialysis should be considered part of supportive care if the patient fits any of the following criteria:

CRITERIA

Stage 3 or 4 coma or hyperactivity caused by dialyzable drug which cannot be treated by conservative means

Hypotension threatening renal or hepatic function which cannot be corrected by adjusting circulating volume

Marked hyperosmolality which is not due to easily corrected fluid problems

Severe acid base disturbance not responding to therapy

Severe electrolyte disturbance not responding to therapy

Marked hypothermia or hyperthermia

IMMEDIATE DIALYSIS INDICATED REGARDLESS OF CLINICAL CONDITION

ethylene glycol - if acidotic start ethanol, then dialyze (see drug list)
methanol - if acidotic start ethanol, then dialyze (see drug list)
heavy metals in soluble compounds
heavy metals after chelating

DIALYSIS INDICATED ON BASIS OF CONDITION OF PATIENT

| alcohols | calcium | potassium |
| ammonia | chloral hydrate | quinidine |

272

amphetamines	fluorides	quinine
anilines	iodides	salicylates
antibiotics	isoniazid	strychnine
barbiturates (long)	meprobamate	thiocynates
boric acid	(Equanil, Miltown)	
bromides	paraldehyde	

Amphetamines respond better to acid diuresis BUT
if not responding, then consider dialysis

While the long acting (renal cleared) barbiturates
are more readily dialyzable than the short
(hepatic cleared), dialysis may be helpful if the
patient has criteria for supportive dialysis needs.

Salicylates generally respond well to the intensive therapy but if complications such as renal
failure develop, peritoneal dialysis with 5% albumin is helpful

Peritoneal dialysis and exchange transfusion may be
more useful in small children than hemodialysis. Again,
the main point of these procedures may be not just for
removal of poison but restoration of fluid or acid base
balance. The infant who has been poisoned and whose
serum sodium is rising because of all the bicarb pushes
may be helped considerably by an exchange even if
little poison is removed.

DIALYSIS IS NOT INDICATED EXCEPT FOR SUPPORT IN THE
FOLLOWING POISONS: THERAPY IS INTENSIVE SUPPORTIVE CARE

antidepressants (tricyclic and MAO inhibitors also)	hallucinogens
antihistamines	Heroin and other opiates
chlordiazepoxide (Librium)	Methaqualone (Quaalude)
digitalis and related	Noludar (Methyprylon)
diphenoxylate (Lomotil)	Oxazepam (Serax)
ethchlorvynol (Placidyl)	Phenothiazines
glutethimide (Doriden)	Synthetic anticholinergics and belladonna compounds

Glutethimide will be found in the dialyzable portion of many lists. It is doubtful that oil dialysis can remove an appreciable quantity. Resin hemoperfusion or charcoal hemoperfusion, new techniques, have been reported to remove them quickly, but the techniques are still questionable because of the large volume of distribution. Conservative therapy provides over 99% salvage and dialysis would only be useful if fluid or electrolyte complications arise.

Dialysis, except in the case of the immediate list, should NOT be performed as initial therapy. Only when the criteria listed on the previous page are met should it be considered.

CHARCOAL PERFUSION

This new device available from Bectin-Dickinson Co. is a method of removing drugs early in the course of an intoxication and may be effective with the drugs on the above list which are not dialyzable. It may also be of assistance with other drugs.

(This drug list is taken from POISINDEX: A computer Generated Emergency Poison Management System. It is copyrighted but may be quoted if prior permission is obtained)

ACTIVATED CHARCOAL - NOT universal antidote which is worthless. NOT antiflatus tablets which are also worthless. NORIT-A or comparable finely divided act-tivated charcoal should be available. 5 to 10 times the estimated dose of the ingested substance should be given. A dose of 15 to 30 grams in an unknown would be acceptable. It can be mixed in a water slurry and drunk or passed down an orogastric tube. A palat-able mixture which has long shelf life is made as follows: 30 grams of activated charcoal and 120 ml water kept in a dark widemouth 6 oz bottle. 7 ml of cherry syrup may be added just before use to provide flavoring. It has a syrupy consistency and should be shaken before use.

AMMONIUM CHLORIDE - 75 mg/kg/dose IV, four times a day to a maximum of 2 to 8 grams per day. May be given orally or intravenously, for urine acidification to pH 4.5 to 5.5. Care should be excercised if the patient is in liver or renal failure.

ANALEPTICS - Coramine, Metrazol, Nikethamide, Bemegride, Doxpram, etc. These agents are SPECIFICALLY CONTRAIN-DICATED IN ALL TOXICOLOGY, regardless of the PDR.

APOMORPHINE - DO NOT USE THIS AGENT UNLESS A NARCOTIC ANTAGONIST IS AVAILABLE. DOSE - 0.1 mg/kg IV or Sub-Q. DO NOT REPEAT. Give copious oral fluids. METHOD - A 6 mg tablet is usually available. Tablets are unsterile. Prepared solutions have very short shelf life and should NOT be kept. The tablet must be crushed and placed in a syringe. The plunger is then replaced and sterile diluent drawn up. For a child 3 cc of diluent are used so that the final concentration is 2 mg/ml. For an adult 1 or 2 cc may be used if the solution is to be given Sub-Q. Time to emesis is 5 to 15 minutes. DO NOT REPEAT. A narcotic antago-nist should be given after emesis has occurred. Narcan (naloxone) is preferable at usual adult dose of 0.4 mg IV or pediatric dose of 0.1 mg IV. NOW ABANDONED BY MOST POISON EXPERTS BECAUSE OF EXCESSIVE AND PROLONGED COMA AND DEPRESSION.

ASCORBIC ACID - 500 mg to 1 gm slowly IV or orally for urine acidification to pH 4.5-5.5 may be repeated as needed.

ATROPINE - In organophosphate poisonings a test dose of 2 mg IV is standard. A test dose in a child should be 0.5 mg/kg. If the patient is indeed poisoned, he will not develop any signs of atropinism and the dose may have to be raised and repeated frequently. The endpoint is stopping secretions NOT just dilation of pupils.

BAL - 3-5 mg/kg/dose every 4 hours IM the first 2 days then 2.5 to 3 mg/kg/dose IM every 6 hours for 2 days then 2.5 to 3 mg/kg/dose every 12 hours for a week IM. Urticaria may respond to Benadryl. Hyperpyrexia may be observed and blood pressure should be monitored.

BENADRYL - For phenothiazine extrapyramidal effects use 2.5 to 5 mg/kg/dose with a maximum single IV dose of 50 mg.

CASTOR OIL - Avoid using this agent as lipoid pneumonia from aspiration is a major problem. Other non-oil cathartics are superior.

CYANIDE ANTIDOTE PACKAGE (Eli Lilly) - Follow instructions sequentially packed with drugs in the kit. Amyl nitrite should be breathed 30 seconds of each 60 seconds. Amyl nitrite MUST be exchanged yearly. Pediatrics: A NOTE SHOULD BE AFFIXED IN AT LEAST 2 places stating the following: Sodium nitrite 10 mg/kg STAT and 5 mg/kg in 30 minutes for pediatrics. 1.65 ml/kg of 25% solution of sodium thiosulfate should then be given. If a child weighs 25 kg or more than adult dose may be given. For adults the entire ampoule of sodium nitrite is given, if this large amount was given to a child fatal methemoglobinemia could result. The chart below relates dosage of sodium nitrite to the child:

Hemoglobin	Initial Dose 3% Sodium Nitrite ml/kg	Initial Dose 25% Sodium Thiosulfate ml/kg
8 grams	0.22 ml (6.6 mg)	1.10 ml
10 grams	0.27 ml (8.7 mg)	1.35 ml
Normal child		
12 grams.......	0.33 ml (10/mg)..........	1.65 ml
14 grams	0.39 ml (11.6 mg)	1.95 ml

Cyanide toxicity may occur and last several hours so
that patients should be treated if exposure has been
documented.

DEFEROXAMINE - 15 mg/kg/hr IV to a total of 90 mg/kg
over 8 hours, as a drip. 90 mg/kg IM once per 8 hours.
Blood pressure should be closely observed. Orally or
for lavage dissolve 5 grams in each liter of lavage
solution and be sure that there is at least 45 mEq of
bicarb/liter of lavage.

DEXAMETHASONE - For cerebral edema 0.1 mg/kg IV or IM
every 4 hours. It is given in pharmacologic amounts
so that a 2-year-old would receive 2 mg IV to start
and 1 mg every 4 hours. If it is stopped in 48 or 72
hours no taper is needed. If used for a Drano ingestion over a 3-week time course, then a taper should be
done.

DOPAMINE - See Vasopressors

D-PENICILLAMINE - 100 mg/kg/day for 5 days on a empty
stomach to a maximum of 1 gram total dose per day.
However, in adults, 500 mg every 6 hours the first day
then 250 mg every 6 hours the second day, then 250 mg
every 8 hours until no further chelation. (e.g., stop
when arsenic falls below 50 mcg excreted per 24 hours
total). Avoid in patients with penicillin allergy,
monitor proteinuria and administer 25 mg pyridoxine
each day.

EDTA - Use CaEDTA NOT NaEDTA (except in special circumstances such as digoxin poisoning). 50 mg/kg/24
hours in 3 divided doses for up to 5 days IV or IM.
Allow at least 2 days in between courses. Maximum
dose is 1 gm/15/kg/day. Urinary excretion as compared
to baseline should be monitored to see if chelation is
productive. Stop when urine returns to nontoxic levels.
Complications are mostly renal tubular necrosis so
fluids must be at least maintenance and should be IV

at first. DO NOT delay institution of therapy more
than 3 hours to obtain urine flow. If diuretics will
not produce urine and adequate fluids have been given,
then chelation followed by hemodialysis should be considered. This is especially true in a child with ANY
symptoms.

ETHANOL - As a 50% sterile vial, 100% sterile vial or
10% IV bottle with glucose. All of these should be
available. Indicated in methanol or ethylene glycol
intoxication. First dose should be 1.0-1.5 ml/kg of
100% solution followed 4 hours later by the same dose.
The goal is to have blood alcohol at 100 mg% and the
dose may have to be increased or dripped continuously.
Constant monitoring of the blood ethanol is crucial.
Glucose must be included in the IV to control hypoglycemia. After good levels are obtained ethanol levels
should be measured every 6 to 8 hours. This level
should be maintained for 3 to 5 days in an ethylene
glycol and 1 to 2 days in a methanol.

IPECAC - Syrup (NOT Elixir)
        ADULT - 30 cc orally
        CHILD - 15 cc orally may repeat at one time
        After the dose is given: PUSH FLUIDS - 8 ounces
        in a child, 16 ounces for adult
                        AMBULATE
                        STIMULATE PHARYNX

ISUPREL - see vasopressors

KAYEXALATE - ADULT dose is 15 grams orally or rectally
1 to 4 times per day as needed with close monitoring
of potassium levels and EKG. PEDIATRIC dose is
1 gram of the resin per milliequivalent of excess
potassium either orally or rectally with close monitoring NOTE: Very high in sodium so monitor sodium
and observe for congestive failure which it may
precipitate.

LEVARTERENOL - see vasopressors

MAGNESIUM SULFATE - 5-20 grams ORALLY or 50-200 cc of
a 10% solution or 10-40 cc of a 50% solution usually
found on the obstetric wards. Children should receive
250 mg/kg with a maximum of 5 grams orally. All
cathartics are given orally. Avoid in renal failure,
use sodium sulfate or sorbitol.

MANNITOL - 1.5 gm/kg in 20% solution IV to maintain
diuresis. Maximum of 100 grams per day. Usually
adults are given 25 grams IV to start, IV rapidly.

METARAMINOL - see vasopressors

METHLENE BLUE - 0.2 ml/kg IV over 5 minutes of a 1%
solution.

MINERAL OIL - Avoid using this agent as lipoid pneumonia from aspiration is a major problem. Other
non-oil cathartics are superior.

NALORPHINE (NALLINE) - Should only be used if Naloxone
is not available. 0.1 mg/kg dose to a maximum of 5
every 30 to 45 minutes. This drug will cause respiratory depression on its own and will augment respiratory
depression produced by barbiturates and other sedatives.
This comes in 5 mg and 0.2 mg vials. PICK CAREFULLY.

NALOXONE (NARCAN) - 5 micrograms/kg/dose (0.005 mg/kg/
dose as needed for reversal. Usual adult dosage is
0.4 mg - 0.8 mg, usual dose in a 2-year-old would be
about 0.1 mg. This does not have any respiratory depressant effect of its own. This agent is far superior to Nalline. Has a short half-life so be prepared
to administer at 30-60 minute intervals especially
with methadone and Darvon.

2-PAM (PROTOPAM, PRALIDOXIME) - For use in organophosphate ingestions AFTER atropine. Must be used within

24 hours of exposure.
Contraindicated in carbamate insecticide exposures
(Sevin, Carbaryl).
Adult dose is 1 gram IV at a rate of 500 mg/minute
(i.e., 2 minutes) and may be repeated every 8-12
hours as needed.
Pediatric dose is 250 mg/dose slowly IV repeated
every 8-12 hours.

PHYSOSTIGMINE SALICYLATE (Antilirium)
Indications - Anticholinergic findings plus hypertension, hallucinations, coma, convulsions, and
arrythmia. Repeat doses should be given only if
life threatening symptoms recur and it must be given
over 60-120 seconds to avoid iatrogenic convulsion.

Contraindications - Asthma, diabetes, urinary ob-
struction present relative contraindications. If
the situation warrants use, have atropine ready at
1/2 dose to reverse physostigmine cholinergic crisis.

PEDIATRIC DOSE

Therapeutic Trial: 0.5 mg slowly intravenously.
If toxic effects persist and no cholinergic effects
are produced, the drug should be readministered
at 5 min. intervals until maximum.

Therapeutic Dose: The lowest total effective trial
dose should be repeated if life threatening signs
recur. Physostigmine is metabolized within 30-60
min. and repeated doses may be necessary. Atropine
should be ready at 1/2 the dose of physostigmine.

ADOLESCENT & ADULT DOSE

Therapeutic Trial: 2 mg IV slowly over 60 seconds.
A second dose of 1-2 mg may be attempted in 20
min. if no reversal has occurred. Monitor EKG
and watch for QRS.

Therapeutic Dose: 1-4 mg IV slowly over 60 seconds. Repeat as life threatening symptoms recur. Physotigmine is metabolized within 30-60 min. and repeated doses may be necessary. Atropine should be ready at 1/2 dose.

SODIUM SULFATE - 250 mg/kg/dose orally for cathartic effect.

SORBITOL - Used as a cathartic 50-100 cc

VASOPRESSORS - It is best to avoid vasopressors and use fluids for hypotension if at all possible. If fluids fail after a reasonable trial, the following may help.

Isuprel - (Isoproterenol - 2 mg in 1000 cc of D_5W makes a concentration of 2 micrograms/ml. Start at 0.1 mcg/kg/min and slowly increase. STOP at a heart rate of 180 to 200.

Levarterenol - (Levophed) - 4 ml vial added to 1000 cc of D_5W to make a solution of 4 micrograms/ml. Use flow rate of 0.1 to 0.2 mcg/kg/min to start and increase as needed.

Metaraminol - (Aramine, Pressonex) - 10 mg/ml in a 10 ml vial. Add 100 mg to 1000 cc of D_5W to make 100 mcg/ml solution. Run at 5 mcg/kg/min to start and increase slowly to obtain desired effect.

Dopamine - 40 mg/cc in 4 cc ampoules. Add 1 ampoule (200 mg) to 250 cc D_5W resulting in 0.8 mg (800 mcg) per cc. Start at 5-10 mcg/kg/min and increase as necessary to 20 mcg/kg/min. Rates in excess have been used but renal shutdown may occur and therefore do not use above 20 mcg/kg/min for prolonged periods.

VETERINARY TOXICOLOGY FOR PHYSICIANS, NURSES, AND PHARMACISTS

Frederick W. Oehme, D.V.M., Ph.D.
*Professor of Toxicology, Medicine and Physiology,
Comparative Toxicology Laboratory, Kansas State
University*

While the Emergency Room and Poison Control Center
are heavily oriented toward human intoxications, a
significant number of inquiries received by these
facilities involve actual or potential animal intoxications. Since animals differ from humans not only in
obvious outward characteristics, but also in physiologic
and biochemical makeup, the extrapolation of recommendations for humans to use in dogs, parakeets, horses,
sheep, or hamsters is often difficult, usually somewhat
complicated, and in some cases downright impossible.
It is often most appropriate to request the opinion of
a veterinary toxicologist when such situations arise;
however, this is not always possible, and it is useful
for the Emergency Room or Poison Control Center personnel to have some acquaintance with the variety and
characteristics of poisonings observed in domestic
animals. The purpose of this paper is to offer the
interested health scientist some insight into the wide
world of Veterinary Toxicology.

The anatomical differences between pets, livestock,
and man are obvious. Coupled with differences in
structure are physiological differences in organ size
and function, and in capacity and limitations of tissue
activity. Differences are also found when the biochemistry of individual tissues and animals are examined.
Enzyme capabilities in digestive tract function, metabolism, and biotransformation systems in the liver, and
transport and other enzymatic processes throughout the
body differ markedly from species to species and between
domestic animals and man. Indeed, the occurrence of

282

these variations is the basic for the entire group of
comparative sciences (1-5).

Of almost equal disease-producing significance with
the anatomical, physiological, and biochemical differences are the effects of domestication and the resulting
characteristics that the animal population have developed
through the years of close affiliation with man. Animals
have become almost entirely dependent upon man for providing the essentials of proper nutrition, housing, and
total environment. Domestic animals have essentially
become creatures of habit and have maintained the specific feeding, grazing, watering, and daily routine
habits that man has imposed. Irregularities in diets
and routine produced by mismanagement leave the animals
with little alternative. They thus have become subject
to man's whims, his attempts to become efficient or to
"cut corners", and also to his stupidity and errors.
The domestic animal is forced to feed and be housed
where man wills. Feed, water, and therapeutic or
prophylactic application of chemicals make animals susceptible to errors in dosages, feed ingredients, faulty
applications of chemicals, and other general mismanagement, with the potential for toxicity always present.

With such a wide variety of potential sources of
error due to animals' complete lack of independence
and total acceptance of their environment, it is common
to find chemical poisonings occurring under wide circumstances. The epidemiological pattern of animal
poisonings is closely related to man's ability to
properly manage his pets and livestock. The following
are examples of some of the common animal poisonings
and reflect the variety and importance of this area.

DRUGS AND HOUSEHOLD PRODUCTS

Errors in the choice of a therapeutic compound, in
its route or mechanism of application, and in its
dosage are common lapses of judgment that result in

poisoning. The faulty selection of a worming preparation, the administration of a new chemical by an other-
than-recommended route of administration, and the overdosage of an anesthetic are dangerous and frequently
fatal errors. Administering a common anthelmintic to
control hookworms in dogs that are debilitated, stressed
or maintained at environmental temperatures higher than
usual has resulted in dramatic fatal reactions (6).
The mistaking of propylene glycol for mineral oil and
the administration of 1 gallon of the wrong material
to horses has resulted in a characteristic toxic reaction
(7). Not only are such errors subject to frank poisoning,
but adverse reactions and a multitude of possible acute
and chronic variations may also occur.

Household chemicals are a popular source of human
poisonings. This is also becoming common in veterinary
medicine due to the increased number and diversity of
chemicals found and used in the home. Asperin, vitamin
and mineral pills, birth control tablets, marijuana
and drugs of abuse, disinfectants, and germicides are
only a few of such hazardous materials (7,8). Because
types of household pets vary from birds through rodents
to dogs and cats, a wide variation in toxic response
is possible. Hence, owners used to exposing their
previous pets to the usual household chemicals, may
find toxicities developing upon the introduction of
a new species of household animal. The phenolic disinfectants are one group of commercial compound for
which this species variation is potentially of importance.

Fig. 1 illustrates the normal phenolic components of
urine from four different animals. The wide variation
in phenol metabolites is obvious and reflects the
variability in ability to detoxify phenolic materials.
Fig. 2 is the plasma disappearance of radioactive
phenol in cats, dogs, pigs, and goats following the
intravenous administration of identical single doses.
The pig and goat demonstrate the ability to rapidly

detoxify and eliminate phenol from the blood. This represents not only liver metabolism, but also excretion, primarily via the kidneys. The dog is intermediate in its rate of plasma clearance, while the cat has a relatively slow capability of removing the toxic phenol from the plasma. As long as the plasma level of the toxic chemical remains high, toxicity is a potential problem. It would further be expected that pigs and goats have little potential for phenol poisoning, dogs would have an average potential for toxicity, and cats would be presented with a greater hazard from exposure to phenolic materials (9-11).

If dogs and cats are exposed to similar doses of pehnolic compounds and their survival time measured, cats respond with greater toxicity than dogs. Dogs are more capable of excreting the toxic phenolic material than cats (10-12). Thus, the capacity of dogs to metabolize and excrete the phenolic compounds is apparently related to that species' ability to withstand doses lethal to cats. Although this species difference has been experimentally demonstrated for a wide variety of household chemicals (aspirin, cleaning fluids, petroleum products, insecticides, disinfectants), the phenolic dosages used to document this effect were greatly in excess of the household exposure to which pets are subjected under usual conditions of household use.

Nevertheless, were it not for man's faulty judgment in applying such compounds directly to and around our domestic animals, toxicities due to errors in selection of the chemical, application route, dosage, or species difference ("I think I'll bathe my cat with this new shampoo; it worked so well on my dogs last year!"), the incidence of poisoning due to drugs and household products would be greatly reduced.

PESTICIDES

This group of chemicals includes insecticides, rodenticides, herbicides, and fungicides; the latter two have the least potential for toxicity. The newer herbicides and fungicides are in general relatively safe, and only the use of some of the older more toxic chemicals are exposure to organic solvents used to carry the chemicals in their application are likely to produce poisoning.

However, rodenticides are an important group of chemicals causing animal poisonings. Strychnine is probably the most common cause of poisonings in dogs and is frequently used to "cleanse" the neighborhood of undesirable dogs (6,8,13-15). The fact that syrychnine can be purchased under the guise of rodent bait greatly increases the hazard of poisoning. Other compounds used for rodent control are at least equally toxic, but the limited distribution of such materials as 1080 (sodium monofluoracetate), ANTU (alphanaphthyl thiourea), phosphorus, metaldehyde, and red squill makes incidence of their toxicity much less than that of strychnine. Warfarin is a readily-available compound used to control rats and mice, but toxicity is limited by the necessity for repeated dosages to be ingested before poisoning usually occurs.

The insecticides are a much more complicated and diverse group of foreign compounds (14,15,17). As causes of animal poisonings, the chlorinated hydrocarbons and the organophosphorus and carbamate materials are hazardous. Fortunately, effective treatments are available for the organophosphorus and carbamate compounds; the chlorinated hydrocarbons are less effectively treated. The widespread use of insecticides around large and small animals results in considerable hazard to these species. Poisoning usually occurs from accidental exposure via spray drift or due to the intentional application of the insecticide to

control livestock or pet insects. In the latter
instance, toxicity may result from improper dilution
of the concentrated material or too frequent application
of acceptable amounts. Both problems are diminished
by users properly reading the labels of the respective
products and abiding closely by the specified recommendations.

Many of the pesticides are capable of accumulating
in feed or food supplies following their application
to the environment. Hence, the widescale use of
insecticides to animals on pasture may result in hay
or feedstuffs growing on neighboring fields developing
residues of these foreign chemicals. Likewise, if
proper precautions in marketing the exposed cattle are
not followed, the meat and by-products from such animals
may contain high residues of the applied chemicals.
Such matters are of vital interest to governmental
regulatory agencies and provide a significant concern
in their efforts to protect not only animal, but also
human health (17).

The government's concern with the accumulation of
foreign compounds in foods and the general environment
has resulted in restrictions on the use of many of the
pesticides. Foremost in such action was the recent
banning of DDT from routine usage in the United States.
This has been followed by other chlorinated hydrocarbons
being examined as a preliminary for similar restrictions.
Many of the rodenticides (strychnine, 1080, ANTU, warfarin), and some of the heavy metal materials used as
herbicides and fungicides, are being re-evaluated by
regulatory agencies because of their hazard and adverse
environmental impact.

HEAVY METAL TOXICANTS

Heavy metals are common factor in producing animal
poisonings because of their wide distribution and use
as agricultural chemicals, components of greases and

oils used on farm machinery, portions of waste materials found in garbage disposed on animal pastures,
their presence in paints and as feed additives, and
the ever-present possibility of their being present
in environmental pollution circumstances. In addition
to their abundance, these compounds have the added
hazard of being persistent in nature; hence their
application to environmental areas and surfaces results
in their being present for many years. Such problems
have been demonstrated by attempts of livestockmen to
dispose of arsenic, lead, and mercury-containing materials by burning or dumping on open ground. The introduction of livestock to such areas in later years has
resulted in severe animal losses.

Lead

Among the variety of heavy metal chemicals potentially
toxic to animals, lead is one of the most frequent
causes of poisoning (7,8,14,15). It is the most common
toxicant in cattle and is available through the ingestion of paint, lead solder or battery terminals, building materials, and various lead-containing sprays. The
poisoning is usually acute and neurological in effect.
Blindness, incoordination, and severe convulsive seizures are observed in affected animals. As cattle
become older, the lead toxicity is usually expressed
as a chronic syndrome with the convulsive pattern less
pronounced. Although acute cases are treated successfully with chelating agents (calcium EDTA), the identification of a lead source for the clinical outbreak
is a valuable diagnostic aid for the puzzled veteri-
narian. Adult cattle with lead poisoning respond well
to removal from the source, good nutrition, and nursing
care.

This toxicity also occurs in dogs and zoo animals
and appears to parallel the occurrence of environmental
pollution, especially that found in heavily polluted
air situations (19). The clinical signs in dogs are

more chronic than that observed in cattle and frequently
are first noticed as a mild gastrointestinal disturbance.
This then progresses to sporadic convulsions easily
confused with epilepsy. After several weeks, affected
dogs may have several convulsive seizures daily. Of
interest is the marked red blood cell changes associated
with this canine toxicity. Anemia, basophilic stippling,
and associated change in physiological function are
seen in some 90+% of dogs affected with lead toxicity
(19). In zoo animals the toxicity is often unobserved
until unexplained deaths occur. Postmortum examination
and chemical analysis of tissues has incriminated lead
in many of these circumstances.

The widespread occurrence of lead has resulted in
studies investigating the behavioral effects of this
heavy metal. Recent studies have demonstrated that
sheep chronically exposed to low levels of lead do
exhibit behavioral and neurological alterations (20).
This observation adds further substance to similar
conclusions drawn in humans and supports the wide
interest in eliminating or reducing lead as an environmental contaminant that is hazardous for all varieties
of animal life. The use of domestic and laboratory
animals are models for studies of lead toxicity has
also been proposed (21). Certain species have been
found to be excellent models if variations due to
differences in physiology and biochemistry are recognized.

Arsenic

Arsenic is a less-frequent intoxication, but very
dramatic when observed. It results from the topical
application or oral absorption of arsenic-containing
insecticides or orchard sprays, as well as consumption
of ant and roach baits. Severe gastrointestinal irritation results in all affected animals, with a bloody
diarrhea common. Deaths are acute. Treatment in the
early stages with BAL (2 mg/lb) every 4 hours and the

application of digestive tract protectants is useful.
An organic form of arsenic, arsenilic acid, is used
as a feed additive for swine. Toxicity results if
feed levels greater than 250 ppm are fed for several
weeks (14), incoordination with posterior ataxia
leading to paresis is seen. Interestingly, appetite
and alterness of the affected animals are normal.
Removal of the swine from the feed source largely
results in progressive recovery.

Copper

The addition of copper to feed rations and supple-
ments has also contributed to poisonings in sheep
and swine. Because of the intentional inclusion of
copper, but the omission of molybdenum in livestock
rations, the resulting biological imbalance produces
a characteristic toxicity (22,23). While the ingestion
of copper (and even the sporadic worming with copper
sulfate in sheep) leads to chronic accumulation of
copper in the system, the signs of poisoning are
acute and lead to death 36-72 hours after onset.
Icterus and hemoglobinuria may be observed, but
usually the animals are "just found dead". The necropsy examination is characteristic of a hemolytic
crisis--generalized icterus, dark metallic-colored
kidneys, swollen friable liver, and a bladder with
brown-black urine (24). The blood is watery and
often fails to clot normally. Treatment is to correct
the copper-molybdenum dietary ratio by spraying 100 mg
ammonium molybdate and 1 G sodium sulfate/head/day on
the feed, adding 1 lb sodium molybdate to every 200 lbs
of salt, or applying 4 ounces of molybdenum superphos-
phate/acre to the pastures.

Mercury

Fortunately, mercury poisoning due to fungicide-
treated seed fed swine is now uncommon. Occasionally,
however, old mercury-treated seed may be included in

animal feeds and can then produce toxicity. Mercury
is a potent nephrotoxin and produces nephrosis and
eventually uremia (15). At necropsy the firm shrunken
kidneys are obvious.

Fluoride

An occasional, but when observed, destructive intoxication is that produced by the chronic ingestion of
fluoride salts. Most frequently this results from
industrial effluents deposited on pastures and consumed with the forage. The condition is chronic and
characteristically produces bone, teeth, and hoof
abnormalities (25). Calves may be born with teeth
or bone lesions if the mother were exposed to fluo-
rides during pregancy. Severe cases of fluorosis
will also exhibit a chronic diarrhea difficult to
differentiate from other intestinal afflictions. No
effective treatment is available, but the addition
of aluminum to the diet will reduce the absorption of
fluoride from the digestive tract.

FERTILIZERS

The problem of synthetic materials, such as nitrates
and ammonia, and also naturally occurring organic
material, such as manure, contributing to animal
poisonings may seem remote. Unfortunately, synthetic
and natural fertilizers are an important cause of
livestock toxicoses. The most obvious situation results from the excessive use of nitrate-containing
fertilizers on crops and the accumulation of high
nitrate levels in the harvested product. These nitrate concentrations in animal feeds can produce
acute or chronic nitrate intoxication and widespread
economic loss. Even the application of manure to
fields can result in high levels of nitrates developing in plants growing in such areas. Not only do
cash crops accumulate toxic levels of nitrate, but
certain weeds, such as pigweed (Amaranthus retroflexus),

are capable of building up heigh levels of nitrate in their organic matrix when grown on soils containing concentrations of nitrates or nitrate-releasing organic matter (7,14,15,26).

An instance of a vacant feedlot that had grown a lush crop of weeds and was used to provide green pasture for cattle illustrates this problem. Within a few hours after a large group of feeder cattle were turned into the weed-covered feedlot, the owner found 17 cattle dead and numerous others in various stages of toxicity. Even though the cattle were promptly removed from the lot, approximately one-third of the animals died from nitrate poisoning. Analysis of the weeds growing in the area revealed concentrations of nitrate as high as 4.5%.

A complicating situation is the relationship between adverse growing conditions and the accumulation of nitrates in plant materials. Although levels of nitrate may be moderate in the soils supporting grain crops (particularly corn or sorghum) or a variety of weeds, under the influence of a drought or the application of plant hormone herbicides, these commonly grown plants may accumulate excessively high and toxic concentrations of nitrate (26,27). The widescale losses in the middle 1950's due to livestock consuming drought-affected corn and sorghum was largely due to nitrate toxicity. The application of 2,4-D to weeds frequently permits these plants to develop transient toxic concentrations of nitrate; if consumed during this temporary phase, nitrate poisoning may result (26).

NATURAL TOXINS

Toxicoses due to plants and animals are not usual in man, but livestock and pet poisonings due to a variety of poisonous plants or toxic venoms are a significant part of veterinary toxicology (4,7,8,26,

31). The basic factor underlying most plant poisoning problems is mismanagement. Livestock are frequently allowed to graze wide areas of natural range land. When weather conditions are bad, pastures may provide less forage than expected and limited plant material for animal consumption and overgrazing frequently results. Under conditions of repeated overgrazing, naturally occurring desirable pasture grasses die out and weeds, many of them poisonous, take over the range. While such weeds are normally unpalatable, hungry live-stock may be forced to consume them and thereby become poisoned. Although most owners recognized overgrazing and the resulting hunger that results in their animals, mismanagement aggravates the loss of native pasture grasses and speeds the introduction and multiplication of poisonous plants. When owners do not provide sup-plemental feeding for animals on such poor pasture land, the livestock are forced to consume the noxious weeds.

Poisonous Plants

A variety of poisonous plants are available to live-stock and household pets and present hazards to their health. The cyanide-producing forages are the most common cause of animal sicknesses due to plants. Usually the sorghums (Johnson grass, sudan grass, milo) are responsible for losses. In addition, arrow-grass (Triglochin spp.), elderberry (Sambucus spp.), wild cherry (Prunus spp.), and the pits of several common fruits (apple, peach, apricot) contain com-pounds with the potential of releasing cyanide upon ingestion. Toxicities usually result from ignorance on the part of owners who feed such plant materials to their animals or who throw fence-row clippings into pastures to utilize the material for forage. Adverse weather conditions and wilting frequently increase the toxic potential.

Halogeton (Halogeton glomeratus) and black greasewood

(Sarcobatus vermiculatus) are two plants that contain
high levels of oxalic acid in their plant matrix.
Although these plants are only commonly found in the
ranges of western states, the oxalic acid is an extremely potent toxin and upon ingestion combines with
serum calcium or magnesium. The clinical situation
resulting from the sudden drop in the blood level of
calcium and magnesium causes large-scale acute deaths.
The loss of thousands of sheep annually in the Rocky
Mountain area is directly due to the ingestion of one
or both of these poisonous plants (32). Only recently
a loss of several thousand sheep in one herd resulted
in the erroneous claim that the release of experimental
nerve gas had caused their death. Upon detailed examination it was found that owner error had resulted in
the sheep consuming the oxalate-containing plants and
the large-scale deaths. Since the calcium and magnesium oxalate salts formed are excreted in the urine
and become crystalized in the kidney tubules, causing
an inability to pass urine, animals that survive the
acute syndrome commonly develop renal failure.

Locoweeks (Astragalus spp. and Oxytropis spp.) are
other common and characteristic causes of livestock
losses in the western states. The plants are not
usually consumed by livestock but under adverse growing
conditions and inadequate natural forage, cattle, sheep,
and horses may be forced to consume them. Once livestock taste the plants they may develop a like for
their flavor and will then preferentially consume
them, even if other feed is supplied. Although horses
and ruminants may consume locoweeks, horses are much
more sensitive to the toxic principle's effect. Hence,
as in one incident when cattle and horses were grazing
the same pasture, horses develop locoweed poisoning
well before cattle show even the earliest signs of
intoxication (33). The clinical syndrome is one of
weight loss and mental derangement. Animals become
easily aggravated and undergo bizarre temperament
changes. Deaths frequently result from self-inflicted

injuries due to running through fences, falling down
wells, or drowning in ponds or streams. The toxin
has an affinity for the nervous system and characteristic microscopic lesions are detected in the neurons
of the brain (33-35).

Selenium is a chemical found in certain types of
rock and hence specific types of soils (23). Plants
growing on such soils may accumulate levels of selenium
in their plant structure varying from only a few ppm
to several 10,000 ppm. While any plant growing on
soils containing selenium may build up low levels of
this chemical, specific plants, such as poison vetch
(Astragalus spp.) and woodyaster (Xylorrhiza spp.),
have the ability to selectively take up and accumulate
massive amounts of selenium. Some of these plants
(golden-weed, Oonopsis spp. and princesplume, Stanleya
spp., for example) will only grow on soils high in
selenium; hence, they are called "indicator plants",
since they indicate the fact that selenium is present
in the soils on which they are growing. Toxicity due
to selenium will produce various clinical signs,
depending upon the concentration of the chemical in
the consumed plants. Low levels of selenium may result
in weight loss, deformed hooves and hair loss, and the
birth of deformed young. Larger amounts of selenium
cause liver damage. A nervous syndrome, similar to
that seen with locoism, commonly develops if large
amounts of selenium are ingested.

Several other poisonous plants produce such a rapid
death that owners may report only that the animals
were found dead. Waterhemlock (Cicuta spp.) grows in
wet areas and contains the highest toxin concentrations
in chambers just above the roots. Animals become exposed by crushing the plant in the stream in which it
is growing and then consuming the toxin-containing
water, or they may actually consume one or more mouth-
fuls of the plant material. The toxin is so severe
that violent muscle spasms may knock the animal off

its feet and cause death within minutes. Cattle poisoned by waterhemlock have been found with walnut-size pieces of the plant still in their mouths.

Common oleander (Nerium oleander) is not only responsible for sudden animal losses, but has also resulted in several human fatalities. Only a small amount of the plant material or toxin-containing sap is required to produce poisoning. Cases have developed from individuals consuming meats cooked using oleander branches as spits. The toxin affects cardiac function and produces a rapid death in all species of animals.

Cocklebur (Xanthium spp.) is a weed capable of infesting almost any barren ground. It appears in the early spring as one of the first forms of green vegetation. Since the plant is so common, it is fortunate that its most potent state is during the early growth period, but unfortunately this is just when other green vegetation is limited. Cattle and hogs may be browsing pastures when early spring rains produce cocklebur sprouting. The resulting sprouts contain high concentrations of hydroquinone, a potent liver toxin capable of producing massive liver necrosis and death within a few hours. The mature cocklebur plant is not palatable to livestock, but the burrs containing the seeds may sprout in the fall following a warm rain. Hence, poisoning may not only occur in the spring, but also in the fall when sprouting cockleburs again aprovide lush forage for grazing animals.

PETROLEUM PRODUCTS

A variety of oils, greases, benzenes, hydrocarbons, and other petroleum products are used on and around domestic animals. Some are employed directly on machinery to which livestock have access; several are utilized as solvents for sprays and materials applied to animals; others are formulated for application to buildings, and animals lick or otherwise contact the

applied product; or animals may directly consume the
petroleum products by gaining access to storage areas
housing opened containers of these materials. In
certain areas of the United States, oil wells and oil
storage tanks provide the potential for cattle consuming the crude petroleum product. Proper care and
precautions are frequently not taken to assure that
animals are protected from exposure. Incomplete
fencings of crude oil holdings or storage areas may
permit inquisitive cattle to satisfy their curiosity.
Ignorance of the potential toxicity of these products
leads owners to utilize various petroleums directly on
livestock as therapeutic aids.

Petroleum products produce a characteristic sequence
of clinical signs. If applied to the skin, irritation
and thickening commonly results. Photosensitization
is frequent, especially in white-haired or light-
skinned individuals. If consumed by mouth, the petroleum material produces digestive disturbances, may be
inhaled with resulting pneumonia, and after several
days can produce liver, kidney and bone marrow dysfunction. Pregnant animals may abort and a poor-doing
individual, continually losing weight and eventually
dying, is a usual outcome. Poisoning due to petroleum
products is a complicated and varied intoxication.
Its occurrence could largely be prevented by owner
education and by assuring that proper precautions were
taken to prevent animal access to these materials.

POLLUTANTS

The occurrence of air, water, industrial, and other
pollutions are just as much animal hazards as they are
for humans. A good correlation may be observed between
animal and human toxicity problems caused by chemicals
polluting the environment. The animal epidemiology is
frequently identical to that observed for humans (18).

Air pollution usually results from industrial fumes

being released to the atmosphere, and animals in the
vicinity are exposed to sulfur and nitrogen oxides,
heavy metals such as zinc and lead, hydrocarbons, and
various forms of particulate matter. Since most industrial plants are located in suburban and rural areas,
livestock grazing surrounding pastures are increasingly
likely to assume body burdens of these chemicals or to
exhibit biological responses to their inhalation.
Since lead from automobile fumes accumulates in the
heavier portions of the air and in particulate matter,
dogs are more likely to exhibit signs of lead poisoning than are the adult humans living in the same environment.

Water pollution is a special problem for rural areas
utilizing streams and wells as municipal water sources.
This is in contrast to large cities that utilize upland
reservoirs many miles distant from the consuming population. The sewage discharge of upstream communities
and industrial complexes and agricultural enterprises
(feedlots, fertilization) may result in a variety of
toxic materials being present in the water used by a
downstream stockman or community for drinking purposes.
The same waters may enter wells supplying other farm-
steads or communities.

Recent interest in nitrate concentrations in water
supplies has resulted in speculation as to the potential
hazard of the continuous ingestion of low-level nitrate
waters (47,48). Water supplies in the mid-west have
widely varying nitrate concentrations. In one survey,
a significant percentage (28.5%) had levels in excess
of 50 ppm, and 19% had nitrate levels in excess of 70
ppm (49). While the influence of nitrates on animal
and human health has only partially been defined,
there is little doubt that the other foreign chemicals
present in water supplies due to industrial and agricultural pollution are indeed capable of producing
significant toxicity.

Other pollutants can produce toxicities under circumstances that are frequently unique to the situation.
Carbon monoxide is a special problem during winter
weather in animals confined in tightly sealed quarters.
Tractors or improperly vented heating equipment utilized
within such facilities may produce lethal concentrations
of this gas. Antifreeze (ethylene glycol) is a special
problem for dogs and cats because of its sweet taste
(50,51). Consumption of this material when owners
discharge radiators in garages or on the ground results
in toxicity due directly to the glycol or due to glycol
metabolism to oxalate which produces renal failure
through the formation of calcium oxalate crystals. As
with most pollution problems, prevention is a matter
of education and regulation, and prophylactic efforts
are immeasurably more rewarding than the treatment of
poisoned individuals.

TOXICOSES COMMONLY OBSERVED IN VARIOUS ANIMALS

Certain intoxications occur more frequently in
various animal species than others. This is due to
the type of environment in which the specific animals
are kept, the management of those animals, and the
chance of exposure to various chemicals under housing
and environmental conditions. In addition, certain
animal species are more sensitive to various chemicals
than others; for example, cattle are extremely sensitive to lead, while cats are much more likely to be
poisoned by phenol than other species. The individual
asked to offer advice on potential toxicity would be
greatly assisted by an indication of the frequency with
which various poisonings are observed in the various
animal species. While such a listing will necessarily
vary with individual circumstances and the specific
portion of the country involved, a general listing of
the intoxications most commonly observed in domestic
animals is offered.

Companion animals are those species used by man for

recreational or psychological purposes and are usually
housed with or in close proximity to their owner.
These include household pets (commonly referred to as
"small animals") and horses. In addition, some people
maintain exotic animals, including reptiles, amphibians,
fish, and various types of birds. Zoos have a full
range of animal species and are subject to interesting
and often unique intoxications. Domesticated food-
producing animals are a rich source of toxicological
case material, and poisonings in cattle, sheep and
goats, swine, and various forms of poultry continually
occur.

Household Pets

The toxicoses seen in dogs and cats are often dramatic
and resemble the incidence found in humans. Because
of close proximity to the owner, these cases are frequently presented for evaluation and therapy at a
relatively early stage. The following is a listing of
the major groups and specific etiological agents commonly observed to cause poisoning in small animals.

Rodenticides: strychnine, sodium fluoroacetate
(1080), thallium, warfarin, metaldehyde

Insecticides: chlorinated hydrocarbons, organophosphorus compounds, carbamates

Heavy metals: lead, arsenic

Herbicides and fungicides

Poisonous plants: mycotoxins, algae, ivies,
mushrooms

Animal toxins: snakes, toads and lizards, tick
paralysis

Drug reactions: aspirin, anthelmintics, drug

interactions

Environmental contaminants: ethylene glycol, garbage,
    phenols

Horses

This species is usually well protected by man from
foreign chemicals. Toxicoses in horses usually develop
from naturally occurring toxins, unintentional lapses
of judgment, or inappropriate or overzealous drug
therapy by trainers or owners. The following is a
summary of the more common poisonings observed.

Poisonous plants: hepatic cirrhosis, gastroenteritis,
    neurological disorders producing icterus, cyanide-
    containing plants

Insecticides and rodenticides: organophosphorus
    compounds, strychnine

Drug reactions: anthelmintics, tranquilizers,
    analgesics

Snake bite

Cattle

The variable husbandry practices associated with
different geographic locations and types of cattle
result in variation in the common observed poisonings.
In general, dairy cattle are more closely confined
and exhibit insecticide or heavy metal intoxication
most frequently. Beef or range cattle often encounter
poisonous plants or dietary contaminants as the agents
responsible for intoxications. Following is a summary
of the most common toxicoses observed in cattle.

Heavy metals: lead, arsenic, mercury, fluorine,
    molybdenum

Insecticides and herbicides

Nitrate-nitrite, oil, and salt contamination of diet

Poisonous plants: bracken fern, equisetum, sweet
clover, ergot, mycotoxins, fescue, cyanide- and
selenium-containing plants, oak, algae, thiaminases

Sheep and Goats

Since sheep and goats range widely over land that is
otherwise often unusable, poisonous plants are a major
part of the factors producing toxicosis in this species.
The list below summarizes the commonly occurring poisonings.

Poisonous plants: photosensitizers, cyanogenic,
selenium-containing, oxalate-containing, lupine,
death camas, locoweed, larkspur, cicuta, conium,
cocklebur, vetches and laurels, white snakeroot

Insecticides and anthelmintics

Heavy metals: copper, thallium, arsenic, lead

Nitrate, sulfur, fluorine, salt, sodium chlorate

Swine

The close confinement of most pigs and the concentrated feeding schedule results in dietary toxins
producing most of the poisonings. As shown in the
following summary, heavy metal and insecticide poisonings are also frequent.

Salt, coal-tar and petroleum products, nitrate-
nitrite, wood preservations

Heavy metals: mercury, copper, arsenic, lead, zinc,
thallium

Poisonous plants: mycotoxins, cocklebur, pigweed
and nightshade, conium, cicuta, crotalaria,
buttercup, photosensitizers

Insecticides and herbicides

Poultry

The short life span of most commercially raised
poultry and the wide range of environment for wild
birds, results in a great variation in the poisonings
commonly observed in this species. These are listed
below:

Insecticides

Heavy metals: arsenicals, mercury

Poisonous plants: locust, corn cockle, crotalaria,
    oleander, tobacco, nightshade, sprouted potatoes,
    mycotoxins, algae, botulism

Rodenticides

Carbon monoxide

Drugs in feed and water: salt, sulfonamides,
    coccidiostats, fungicides

The Japanese yew (Taxus cuspidata) is an ornamental
plant that recently has been shown to produce acute
poisonings in animals consuming clippings. The plant
is frequently installed around fences and animals may
become exposed to clippings or may browse the plant
directly through the fence. The toxic principle has
not yet been fully defined, but horses and ruminants
have been found dead by amazed owners following access
to this plant (36). Even though oleander and yew are
attractive plants to beautify landscapes around homes
and other structures, their toxicity provide great
hazards not only for pets and livestock, but also for

children accustomed to placing foreign objects in
their mouths.

Perhaps the most subtle and potentially damaging
hazard from plants is that which results from pregnant
animals consuming weeds containing one or more teratogenic principles. Numerous instances of such effects
have been reported and many have been confirmed under
experimental circumstances (37-39). The types of
defects recorded vary from skeletal to soft tissue
alterations and in many cases multiple anomalies are
documented. The study of such occurrences is a vast
field for future research.

Fungal Toxins

Some of the lower members of the plant family, the
fungi, are capable of producing a variety of toxins.
This particular group of poisons, mycotoxins, has
become a focal point for scientific investigation
during the past decade (40). The aflatoxins are a
group of mold poisons produced by specific strains of
the fungi Aspergillus flavus and Penicillium spp. (40).
As with all fungi, a source of nourishment and proper
amounts of moisture and heat must be present to support
growth. Under suitable conditions, these fungi, and
others capable of producing toxins, will grow and in
their growth processes will produce their toxins (41).
Hence, the toxins are products of fungal growth; the
mere presence of the fungus does not necessarily
indicate that its particular toxin is also present.
Conversely, the toxin can be present and viable fungi
may no longer exist in the sample. Mold toxins commonly develop in stored grains and on certain feedstuffs subjected to unusual weathering or storage
conditions. Although moldy feed is usually grossly
identifiable, the spoiled feed may be mixed into a
ration or otherwise offered for livestock consumption
through ignorance or by intention. Animals will
usually reject extremely spoiled feed, but well-diluted

feeds or rations offered hungry cattle may result in acceptance and toxicity.

Most fungal toxins affect the liver and produce lesions varying from frank necrosis to biochemical interference with enzymes or blood-clotting mechanisms. Digestive tract disturbances, photosensitization, poor feed utilization, abortions, and reproductive failures have been also associated with mycotoxin consumption (42). Although cancer has never been associated with clinical instances of mycotoxicoses, the experimental production of tumors by aflatoxins in some laboratory animals has resulted in concern over the concentrations of this toxin in grains destined for human consumption. Only a few of the toxins of potential fungal origin have presently been identified (43). There is no doubt that this interesting area will continue to attract the attention of toxicologists, chemists, and animal scientists for some time to come.

Toxins of Animal Origin

A wide variety of animal-origin toxins are found throughout the world (44,45). However, because of limited accessibility and usual close confinement, only a few toxins produced by animals are hazardous to domestic animals. These intoxications are due to toxins produced by ticks, toads, and snakes. The clinical effects and their resolution are similar to those experienced in humans.

FEED ADDITIVES

The use of chemicals added to livestock rations for the purpose of increasing feed efficiency and reducing disease is a characteristic unique to animal production (46). Although this practice has greatly benefited the livestock economy, the practice is not without danger. Whenever foreign compounds are added to feeds, the possibility of error and resulting animal or human hazard increases. While the presence of chemical residues in human foods and their potential contribution to adverse effects in man is of most concern to public health officials, animals directly consuming feeds containing feed additives are also likely to become grossly toxic. This may be due to improper mixing of the ration, incomplete following of feeding recommendations, faulty husbandry, or mismanagement. In these instances, acute poisonings result from livestock consuming feeds to which they are unaccustomed or because the feed contains unusually high levels of one or more toxic materials (14). Two such common poisonings are those produced by excessive or improper feeding of urea or salt.

The factors frequently associated with the development of urea poisoning in cattle are due to: only roughage being fed before urea was offered; no previous urea being fed; switching to high urea ration suddenly; "bully cattle" getting all the feed; cattle being unusually hungry and overeating; feeding instructions not followed carefully; accidently feeding the wrong mixture; and improper or incomplete feed missing processes. Urea is a protein supplement fed ruminant animals to provide an economical source of protein to the consuming individuals. The production of ammonia from the urea by the ruminal microorganisms is normally followed by incorporation of the ammonia into bacterial protein; this protein is digested in the intestinal tract of the ruminant and serves as a source of nutrient protein. Under conditions of mismanagement the production of ammonia becomes excessive and the rumen microorganisms are unable to utilize the ammonia in its entirety. Ammonia poisoning then results, with the onset of clinical signs within minutes and death frequently following in 1-2 hours.

Salt is a necessary dietary ingredient, but in excess or in the absence of sufficient fresh water it may become toxic. Toxicity occurs most commonly in swine, but also occasionally in cattle, due to a variety of

management factors leading to the accumulation of
sodium ion in the central nervous system and other
body tissues. If the owner then discovers that water
was unavailable to the animals for a period of time,
and then provides unlimited access to water, the
osmotic pressure produced by the sodium results in
increased central nervous system pressure and an acute
neurological and convulsive syndrome. While the condition in cattle is somewhat more chronic and digestive
signs are more prominent, the underlying cause of salt
poisoning is human error resulting in poor animal husbandry practices.

CONCLUSIONS

The variety of foreign chemicals capable of producing animal poisonings is always infinite. As long as such potentially toxic materials exist and are utilized by livestockmen and animal owners, hazards for animals, human and domestic alike, will be a prominent concern. Persons responsible for animal care should be aware of the hazards associated with the use of these chemicals, and they must be instructed and encouraged to use good judgment in their application.

Continuing education is required to avoid user error or ignorance in the exposure of domestic animals to drugs, pesticides, plants and naturally occurring chemicals, and pollutants added to water and food supplies. Individuals with the responsibilities for animal care should recognize their obligation to provide safe environments for their animals and to utilize chemicals appropriately for specified uses. Health personnel dealing with potential or actual poisoning situations in animals also have the obligation to be aware of the variety and general characteristics of animal toxicities. Further, they should recognize the often vast difference between human and animal responses to chemicals and the importance of recognizing species differences when offering prognoses or making recommendations for therapy. A familiarity with the general physiology of the various animal species and an understanding of the type and variety of intoxications that may be expected in the animal kingdom can be most appropriately supplemented by consultations with veterinary clinical toxicologists familiar with the variations that often make the difference between life and death. Common sense and the application of sound basis medical principles are of paramount importance in handling any poisoning, be it in a domestic animal or a human.

REFERENCES

1. Baker C, Tripod J, Jacob J (eds): The problem of species differences and statistics in toxicology. *Proc Eur Soc Study Drug Toxicity, Vol XI.* Amsterdam, Excerpta Media Foundation, 1970.

2. Oehme FW: Species differences: The basis for and importance of comparative toxicology. *Clin Toxicol* 3:5-10, 1970.

3. Oehme FW (ed): Symposium on veterinary toxicology. *Clin Toxicol* 5:141-302, 1972.

4. Oehme FW (ed): Symposium on Comparative toxicology: The relationship between animals and humans. *Clin Toxicol* 7:139-206, 1974.

5. Oehme FW: Comparative toxicology is where it's at... *Clin Toxicol* 7:139-140, 1974.

6. Penumarthy L, Oehme FW, Menhusen MJ: Investigations of therapeutic measures for disophenol toxicosis in dogs. *Am J Vet Res* 36:1259-1262, 1975.

7. Oehme FW: Practical clinical toxicology. *Proc Annual Conf Vet.* Manhattan, Kansas, Kansas State University, 1972.

8. Oehme FW: Clinical toxicology. *Scientific Presentations and Seminar Synopses of the 39th Annual Metting AAHA.* Las Vegas, AAHA, 1972.

9. Oehme FW: *Comparative Study of the Biotransformation and excretion of phenol.* Dissertation, Columbia, University of Missouri, 1969.

10. Oehme FW: Comparative toxicity of 0-phenylphenol and an o-phenylphenol containing disinfectant. *Toxicol Applied Pharmacol* 19:412, 1971.

11. Oehme FW: New Information on the toxicity of phenolic compounds in small animals. *Gaines Newer Knowledge About Dogs* 21:8-15, 1971.

12. Oehme FW, Smith THF: The metabolism and urinary excretion of o-phenylphenol in dogs and cats. *Toxicol Applied Pharmacol* 22:292, 1972.

13. Aronson AL: Chemical poisonings in small animal practice, in *Symposium on Emergencies in Veterinary Medicine. Vet Clin N Amer* 2:379-395, 1972.

14. Buck WB, Oswelier GD, Van Gelder GA: *Clinical and Diagnostic Veterinary Toxicology.* Dubuque, Iowa, Kendall-Hunt Publishing, 1973.

15. Clarke EGC, Clarke JL: *Garner's Veterinary Toxicology,* ed 3. Baltimore, Williams & Wilkins, 1967.

16. Oehme FW (ed): Physical and chemical disorders, in Kirk RW (ed): *Current Veterinary Therapy V: Small animal practice.* Philadelphia, Saunders, 1974.

17. Radeleff RD: *Veterinary Toxicology,* ed 2. Philadelphia, Lea & Febiger, 1970.

18. Miller MW, Berg GG (eds): *Chemical Fallout.* Springfield, Illinois, Charles C. Thomas, 1969.

19. Zook BC: Lead intoxication in dogs. *Clin Toxicol* 6:377-388, 1973.

20. Van Gelder GA, Carson T, Smith RM, et al: Behavioral toxicology assessment of the neurologic effect of lead in sheep. *Clin Toxicol* 6:405-418, 1973.

21. Scharding NN, Oehme FW: The use of animal models for comparative studies of lead poisoning. *Clin Toxicol* 6:419-424, 1973.

22. Buck WB, Ewan RC: Toxicology and adverse effects of mineral imbalance. *Clin Toxicol* 6:459-485, 1973.

23. Underwood EJ: *Trace Elements in Human and Animal Nutrition,* ed 3. New York, Academic Press, 1971.

24. Oehme FW: Copper toxicity in ruminant animals. *Southwestern Vet* 19:295-301, 1966.

25. Shupe JL, Olson AE, Sharma RP: Fluoride toxicity in domestic and wild animals. *Clin Toxicol* 5:195-214, 1972.

26. Kingsbury JM: *Poisonous Plants of the United States and Canada.* Englewood Cliffs, New Jersey, Prentice-Hall, 1964.

27. Hulbert LC, Oehme FW: *Plants Poisonous to Livestock,* ed 3. Manhattan, Kansas, Kansas State University, 1968.

28. Evers RA, Link RP: *Poisonous Plants of the Midwest and Their Effects on Livestock,* Special Publication 24. Urbana, Illinois, University of Illinois College of Agriculture, 1972.

29. Liener IE (ed): *Toxic Constituents of Plant Foodstuffs.* New York, Academic Press, 1969.

30. Schmutz EM, Freeman BN, Reed RE: *Livestock Poisoning Plants of Arizona.* Tucson, University of Arizona Press, 1968.

31. Sperry OE, Dollahite JW, Hoffman GO, et al: *Texas Plants Poisonous to Livestock.* College Station, Texas, Texas A & M University Agricultural Experiment Station, 1968.

32. James LF: Oxalate toxicosis. *Clin Toxicol* 5:231-244, 1972.

33. Oehme FW, Bailie WE, Hulbert LC: *Astragalus mollissimus* (locoweed) toxicosis in horses in western Kansas. *J Am Vet Med Assoc* 152:271-278, 1968.

34. James LF: Syndromes of locoweed poisoning in livestock. *Clin Toxicol* 5:567-574, 1972.

35. Van Kampen KR, James LF: Sequential development of the lesions in locoweed poisoning. *Clin Toxicol* 5:575-580, 1972.

36. Lowe JE, Hintz HF, Schryver HF, et al: *Taxus cuspidata* (Japanese yew) poisoning in horses. Cornell Vet 60:36-39, 1970.

37. Binns W, Keller RF, Balls LD: Congenital deformities in lambs, calves, and goats resulting from maternal ingestion of *Veratrum californicum:* Hare lip, cleft palate, ataxia, and hypoplasia of metacarpal and metatarsal bones. *Clin Toxicol* 5:245-261, 1972.

38. Keller RF: Known and suspected teratogenic hazards in range plants. *Clin Toxicol* 5:529-565, 1972.

39. Leipold HW, Oehme FW, Cook JE: Congenital arthrogryposis associated with ingestion of jimsonweed by pregnant sows. *AM J Vet Med Assoc* 162:1059-1060, 1973.

40. Goldblatt LA (ed): *Aflatoxin.* New York, Academic Press, 1969.

41. Campbell TC, Gurtoo HL, Portman RS, et al: Influence of environmental factors on mycotoxin toxicity as evidenced by studies with aflatoxin. *Clin Toxicol* 5:517-528, 1972.

42. Goldblatt LA: Implications of mycotoxins. *Clin Toxicol* 5:453-464, 1972.

43. Stoloff L: Analytical methods for mycotoxins. *Clin Toxicol* 5:465-494, 1972.

44. Brown JH: *Toxicology and Pharmacology of Venoms from Poisonous Snakes.* Springfield, Illinois, Charles C Thomas, 1973.

45. Minton SA (ed): Symposium on snake venoms and evenomation. *Clin Toxicol* 3:343-512, 1970.

46. National Academy of Sciences: *Use of Drugs in Animal Feeds,* Publication 1679. Washington, DC, NAS-NRC, 1969.

47. Oldon JR, Oehme FW, Carnahan DL: Relationship of nitrate levels in water and livestock feeds to herd health problems on 25 Kansas farms. *Vet Med Small An Clinician* 67:257-269, 1972.

48. Ridder WE, Oehme FW: Nitrates as an environmental, animal, and human hazard. *Clin Toxicol* 7:145-159, 1974.

49. Ridder WE, Oehme FW, Kelley DC: Nitrates in Kansas ground-waters as related to animal and human health. *Toxicology* 2:397-405, 1974.

50. Sanyer JL, Oehme FW, McGavin MD: Systematic treatment of ethylene glycol toxicosis in dogs. *AM J Vet Res* 34:527-534, 1973.

51. Penumarthy L, Oehme FW: Treatment of ethylene glycol toxicosis in cats. *AM J Vet Res* 36:209-212, 1975.

SALICYLATE POISONING

Anthony R. Temple, M.D.
Director, Intermountain Regional Poison Control Center
Associate Professor of Pediatrics, University of Utah
College of Medicine
Associate Professor of Clinical Pharmacology and
Toxicology, University of Utah, College of Pharmacy

I. General Information

A. Incidence

Salicylates are the most important cause of both
accidental ingestions and accidental poisoning
deaths among children under the age of 5 years.
In addition, they are frequently employed by
adults for suicidal purposes, and therapeutic
overdosage is also frequently responsible for
salicylate poisoning.

B. Etiology

1. Most cases of salicylate poisoning involve
the ingestion of aspirin. Among cases of accidental ingestion of salicylates by children,
flavored children's tablets (1 1/4 grain) are
most frequently involved; however, the adults'
tablets (5 grain) are more dangerous because of
the larger quantity of salicylate involved.

2. The most serious cases of salicylate poisoning are those which arise in children from the
therapeutic use of excessive or too-frequent
doses of aspirin over a period of days. For
example, in the author's recent experience such
cases account for 30 percent of 51 aspirin
poisoning cases serious enough to require hospitalization (though they represent only a miniscule

fraction of the total cases), one-third of the
deaths, and have required an average hospitalization of 4 days, compared with 1.7 days for
acute ingestion.

3. While aspirin is the commonest cause of salicylate poisoning, several compounds can cause
similar difficulties. One of the most important
of these is methyl salicylate (oil of wintergreen),
which causes a disproportionately large number of
salicylate poisoning deaths. The great toxicity
of this material is related to the very high
concentration of salicylate, the potentially
lethal dose of oil of wintergreen for a 2-year-
old child being in the range of 1 teaspoon.

4. The toxic effects of aspirin, oil of wintergreen, and also sodium salicylate are qualita-
tively identical, so that the following discussion
applies to poisoning with any of these materials.

5. On the other hand, the aspirin substitutes,
salicylamide and acetaminophen, produce an entirely different type of poisoning.

6. Acetaminophen is available in several products
including Tempra, Tylenol, and Liquiprin.

7. Salicylate poisoning usually results from
ingestion, but percutaneous absorption of salicylates, especially oil of wintergreen, if extensively applied to the skin, has also caused
poisoning on rare occasions.

C. Toxic Dose

1. Although some symptoms of intoxication may
occur at lower doses, severe intoxication is
unlikely to occur in a previously healthy individual with doses of less than about 1 1/2 to 2

grains/pound, or about 200-300 mg/kg.

2. Dehydration, febrile illness, inherently slow metabolism of salicylate or renal dysfunction may be responsible for the development of serious symptoms at lower doses of salicylate.

II. Pathophysiology and Symptoms

A. General Picture

Early symptoms of intoxication, usually related to stimulation of both the central nervous system and metabolism, include vomiting, tinnitus, hyperpnea, confusion (sometimes mania), hyperthermia and generalized convulsions in severe cases. The early stimulatory phase may be followed by varying degrees of depression, ranging from lethargy to frank coma. In fatal cases, death usually occurs during this phase and is related to respiratory failure or cardiovascular collapse.

B. Acid-Base Disturbances

1. Of greatest importance to treatment is the pathogenesis of the acid-base disturbance which may occur, for it poses the most difficult and important therapeutic problem. While the underlying mechanisms have not been defined precisely, the sequence of resulting events is well known, as diagrammed in Figure 1.

2. Hyperpnea is universally present early in the course of salicylate poisoning. It is the result of a direct effect of the salicylate ion upon central control of respiration, producing respiratory alkalosis.

3. The sequence of events of salicylate poisoning is strikingly age-dependent. The acid-base

316

disturbance tends not to progress any further
in adults and in older children; however, other
factors leading to the development of metabolic
acidosis characteristically come into play in
the infant or young child with severe poisoning.

4. Infants and children under the age of about
4 years, and especially those whose poisoning
results from the administration of excessive
aspirin over a period of days, are particularly
susceptible to the development of severe acidosis.

5. Chronic (therapeutic) poisoning is especially
difficult to treat, has a high mortality rate and
causes a progressively increasing percentage of
the deaths from salicylate poisoning (as severe
acute poisonings have declined in incidence).

6. The evolution of the acid-base equilibrium
disturbances can be diagrammed as in Figure 2.
This is a graphic presentation of the Henderson-
Hasselbalch equation relating blood pH, carbon
dioxide (or bicarbonate) content, and carbon
dioxide tension (pCO_2).

7. The events enumerated occur simultaneously,
so that infants and children with severe poisoning usually exhibit evidence of the mixed disturbance, either with a relatively normal blood
pH or frank acidosis at the time of admission.

C. Dehydration

1. Serious dehydration may occur in cases of
severe poisoning because of the combined effects
of hyperpnea, increased insensible water loss
due to hypermetabolism, and the excretion of an
increased solute load.

2. Fluid losses may be as high as 4 to 6 liters/
sq m, especially in young children who have been

poisoned over a period of days. Losses in the vicinity of 2 or 3 liters/sq m are estimated to occur usually.

D. Other Symptoms

1. Depletions of total body sodium and potassium occur inevitably in cases of severe poisoning (unless complicated by renal failure).

   a. Hyponatremia or hypernatremia may occur in infants and young children, depending upon the relative losses of salt and water and the nature of the fluid intake of the patient.

   b. Critical degrees of hypokalemia have been reported in adult patients who develop frank respiratory alkalosis of long duration.

2. Mild and transient hyperglycemia and glycosuria are common and of no clinical significance; however, hypoglycemia of a life-threatening degree may occur, especially in infants.

3. Hemorrhagic complications may result either from a relatively specific inhibitory effect of salicylate upon prothrombin production or, less commonly, as a result of thrombocytopenia or other coagulation defects.

4. Transient renal failure is a relatively rare complication.

5. Oliguria mimicking renal failure may also occur as a result of inappropriate ADH secretion, hyponatremia or inadequate fluid intake.

6. Cerebral edema is not uncommon in very severe cases.

7. Pulmonary edema may develop in those who experience cardiac insufficiency for any of several reasons, including overloading with fluids.

III. Diagnosis and Evaluation

A. General Priniciples

The possibility of salicylate poisoning should be considered in any patient who presents with unexplained hyperpnea in association with vomiting, confusion, lethargy, fever, coma and/or convulsions.

B. Laboratory Tests

1. The ferric chloride test is extremely sensitive and is a useful indicator of the presence of salicylate; however, it has no quantitative value, since strongly positive tests are obtained in patients with relatively small burdens of salicylate. The test is performed by adding a few drops of an approximately 10 per cent solution of ferric chloride to urine; in the presence of salicylic acid, a violet to purple color develops.

2. The definitive diagnostic procedure is the quantitative measurement of salicylate in serum, provided the result is interpreted correctly. The most useful method is the Trinder procedure, which requires only a single reagent with a measured quantity of serum.

3. The serum salicylate level, by whatever means it is measured, can be correlated with the severity of intoxication.

a. The Done nomogram was developed for this purpose and is reproduced in Figure 3.

b. With this nomogram, it is possible to obtain a satisfactory estimate of the expected severity of intoxication on the basis of the blood level of salicylate, provided that the interval since ingestion is known.

c. The usual symptoms exhibited by patients in the various severity classifications shown in the nomogram are:

Asymptomatic. Occasional subjective, but no objective manifestations.

Mild. Mild to moderate hyperpnea, sometimes with lethargy.

Moderate. Severe hyperpnea, prominent neurologic disturbances (marked lethargy and/or excitability) but no coma or convulsions.

Severe. Severe hyperpnea, coma or semicoma, sometimes with convulsions.

The line in the nomogram which bisects the word "severe" indicates the level above which survival is highly unlikely with conventional methods of treatment. This is not meant to imply that fatality may not occur at lower levels, but only to point out the level which probably must be considered to be incompatible with life.

d. It should be emphasized that the nomogram is applicable only to patients who have ingested salicylate in a single dose. In patients who have received salicylate over an extended period of time, the salicylate level bears little relationship to the severity of symptoms, and it becomes necessary to use clinical manifestations as the guage of severity.

e. It is important to be certain that the individual has reached his peak salicylate level
since failure to do so may lead to an under-
estimate of severity. The initial salicylate
level should be obtained after about 6 hours,
and a second value obtained in another 2 to 4
hours to determine that the salicylate level
is declining satisfactorily.

4. Accurate evaluation of the acid-base status is
essential to optimum treatment.

a. Accurate determination of the acid-base status
can be achieved only with measurements of any
two of the following: blood pH, serum or
plasma carbon dioxide content, or the carbon
dioxide tension in blood (pCO_2).

b. If the appropriate determinations for evaluating acid-base status by the means mentioned
above are not available, the presence of
acidosis can be assumed to be present in
children under the age of 4 years who have
severe symptoms and a carbon dioxide content
of less than about 8 mEq/liter, or a CO_2 combining power of less than about 10 mEq/liter,
or in infants subjected to repeated therapeutic
overdosage with aspirin who have had symptoms
of intoxication for more than 24 hours.

c. The urine pH is of no value whatever in defining the acid-base disturbance.

5. In summary, tests which are recommended include,
serum salicylate, blood pH, serum CO_2 (any two),
serum sodium and potassium, blood urea nitrogen or
creatinine, blood glucose, and urine pH and specific
gravity.

IV. <u>Treatment</u>

A. <u>Emptying of Stomach</u>

1. In cases of acute ingestion of a salicylate, early emptying of the stomach is of crucial importance.

2. It has been shown in specific relation to salicylate that induction of vomiting is actually more efficient than is the more laborious and time-consuming gastric lavage, so it is recommended unless the patient is unconscious or having convulsions.

3. Forced (induced) vomiting is more effective than spontaneous vomiting, so administration of an emetic should be done even though the patient has vomited.

4. Emptying of the stomach is best accomplished within 4 hours of the ingestion, although some salicylate can be removed for up to 24 hours.

5. A cathartic may be used to hasten the passage of unrecovered salicylate through the intestinal tract.

6. The oral administration of sodium bicarbonate is contraindicated because it may enhance the absorption of salicylate.

B. <u>Fluid Therapy</u>

1. Mild salicylate poisoning usually can be managed satisfactorily by ensuring an adequate oral intake of fluids, but in more severe cases parenteral fluid therapy is recommended.

2. The recommended plan for parenteral fluid therapy depends upon the acid-base status of the patient and is summarized in the following table. The plan is based upon the opinion and observation that the acid-base disturbance can usually be managed most safely and effectively through adequate hydration with hyptonic polyionic solutions and correction of potassium deficits. (See Table 1).

3. Alkali administration can be expected to produce transient buffering of plasma pH, but persistent correction can be obtained only after fluid and electrolyte (especially potassium) deficits are restored.

C. Symptomatic Measures

1. Therapeutic measures aimed directly at the hyperpnea or prevention of its immediate effects are contraindicated. Respiratory center depressants will decrease the hyperpnea, but unfortunately they also increase the mortality rate, probably because of the need for hyperpnea to provide oxygen sufficient to meet the increased tissue caused by a great increase in the metabolic rate, the latter assumed to be due to uncoupling of oxidative phosphorylation.

2. Respiratory depression may occur and require artificial ventilation with oxygen. It should be remembered that the metabolic rate in salicylate intoxication is greatly increased, such that tissue oxygen requirements and the necessity for elimination of carbon dioxide may be greatly increased. Respiratory stimulants are of no value as a substitute for assisted ventilation inasmuch as maximum respiratory stimulation is already present.

Table 1. Schedule of Intravenous Fluid Administration for Salicylate Intoxication

	Fluid	Rate
Initial hydration	A	400 ml/sq m in 1 hr
If shock present	plasma or blood	10-15 ml/kg in 1 hr, then fluid as for initial hydration
After urine flow established		
Mild or no acidosis	B	2.5-3.5 liter/sq m/24 hr
Severe acidosis	C	3-5 liter/sq m/24 hr
Additional urgent buffering		
of profound acidosis	Na bicarbonate	3-5 mEq/kg in 2-4 hr
		or, if acidosis unresponsive or Na restriction desired
	Tromethamine	3-5 ml of 0.3 M solution in 1 hr
	Determine further needs by blood pH measurement (<7.18)	

COMPOSITION (mEq/liter) AND PREPARATION OF FLUIDS

Fluid	Na	K	Cl	HCO$_3$ or lactate	Preparation
A	75	0	50	25	330 ml 10% dextrose 170 ml normal (0.9%) saline 14 ml 7.5% Na bicarbonate
B	40	35	40	20	"Electrolyte 75", "Isolyte M" or "Butler-Talbot Solution" (as is)
C	55	35	40	35	500 ml Fluid B 8.5 ml 7.5% Na bicarbonate

Further, such drugs may potentiate the convulsant effects of salicylate.

3. For severe convulsions diazepam (2 to 6 mg/sq m slowly) or a short-acting barbiturate may be used intravenously. In rare instances, it may be necessary to resort to general anesthesia to terminate status epilepticus.

4. Tetany may occur, especially during the early phase of alkalosis or else during the period of recovery (in which alkalosis may again occur). It is rarely severe, however, unless alkali therapy is given too rapidly or in excessive amounts. The tetany is due to a diminution in ionized calcium. Slow intravenous administration of calcium (2 to 5 ml of a 10 per cent calcium gluconate solution) is indicated in all patients who develop convulsions. Cessation of the seizures suggests that the problem is one of decreased ionized calcium rather than the direct central effect of potentially lethal amounts of salicylate.

5. Hemorrhagic manifestations may be the result of a variety of coagulation defects, but most commonly are due to a rather specific effect of salicylate in inhibiting prothrombin formation by the liver. This complication can be prevented or reversed by the administration of vitamin K_1 or its oxide intravenously in a dose of 25 to 50 mg. There is merit in routinely treating patients having severe salicylate poisoning with such medications in order to prevent hemorrhagic complications.

6. Hyperpyrexia may occasionally be of sufficient severity to require specific treatment. For this purpose, cautious sponging with tepid water or cooling mattresses are the safest procedures.

7. Renal failure is a rare occurrence in a salicylate poisoning, but is an absolute indication
for the performance of one of the dialysis procedures described below.

D. Artificial Removal of Salicylate

1. Forced diuresis is of limited value since the
rate of excretion of salicylate is not affected
to any appreciable extent by urine volumes in
excess of normal. It is imperative, of course,
that adequate fluid be supplied to ensure normal
renal function (about 25 ml/sq m/hr), however,
beyond that there is little augmentation of
salicylate excretion by increasing urine volumes.

2. The early administration of sufficient quantities
of sodium bicarbonate has been widely advocated
to alkalinize the urine. This form of treatment
is based upon the well-known fact that salicylate
is excreted more rapidly in an alkaline urine.
There is no question that the excretion of
salicylate is markedly accelerated if the urine
can be alkalinized. However, the efficacy of
this approach was suggested by observations on
children who did not, with few exceptions, have
severe intoxication associated with acidosis,
or adults who were alkalotic. The fact of the
matter is that the urine of severely poisoned,
and especially acidotic, patients cannot be
alkalinized even by the administration of
sufficient quantities of bicarbonate without
producing dangerous systemic alkalosis. Alkalinization of the urine is nearly impossible to
achieve in patients having significant potassium
deficits. Consequently, potassium restoration
is essential for alkali administration to alkalinize the urine of patients with severe intoxication. Unfortunately, the rapidity with which
this can be accomplished is restricted by the

limits for the safe parenteral administration
of potassium.

3. Undoubtedly, the most efficient removal of
salicylate from the body is by means of extra-
corporeal hemodialysis (the artificial kidney).
Certainly, in centers where this procedure can
be made available and where there are experienced
hemodialysis teams, it should be used. However,
the procedure suffers from the disadvantages of
requiring a relatively elaborate set-up, not being universally available, requiring extremely
careful laboratory monitoring, being technically
difficult in small children, being time-consuming,
and posing the threat of dangerous blood volume
fluctuations in infants.

4. Peritoneal dialysis offers the advantages that
it is adaptable to almost any hospital setting,
requires less laboratory monitoring, is simple,
relatively safe, and requires little in the way
of equipment. It is less efficient in achieving
a rapid reduction of salicylate level, but can
be continued without interruption for relatively
long periods of time. Because salicylate is
avidly bound to serum proteins, peritoneal
dialysis employing a 5 per cent solution of
human serum albumin, together with the appropriate concentrations of electrolytes, is far
more efficient than the use of protein-free
dialysis solutions. (In the form of commercially
available Albumisol, it is possible to obtain a
solution of 5 per cent human albumin in an
isosmotic buffer which already contains the
necessary quantities of all essential electrolytes with the exception of potassium and calcium.
Thus, one can use this solution simply by adding
potassium chloride in an amount of 5 mEq/liter,
unless renal failure with hyperkalemia is present in which case the potassium is omitted).

5. Exchange transfusion has little or no place in the treatment of salicylate poisoning at the present time because the same thing can be accomplished more quickly and safely with peritoneal dialysis.

6. Hemoperfusion now appears to be another reasonable effective procedure.

V. Chronic salicylism

A. Relative severity

1. Chronic salicylism, while having essentially the same symptoms as those seen in acute poisoning, tends to result in much greater morbidity and mortality. The following table compares hospitalization and death rates in the two types of poisoning:

CONTRIBUTION OF THERAPEUTIC OVERDOSAGE TO
POISONING BY SALICYLATES IN PRE-SCHOOL CHILDREN

	Hospitalizations		Deaths	
	ACC.	THER.	ACC.	THER.
Literature summary (Tainter) 1942-66				
No.	267	193	7	37
%	58	42	16	84
Primary Children's Hospital, SLC, 1967-71				
No.	21	14	0	0
%	60	40	0	100

This data indicates that chronic salicylism is much more likely to result in hospitalization and that deaths from salicylates in children is almost always due to chronic intoxification.

2. Our own experience also indicates that the average length of stay in the hospital is three times as long for chronic salicylism as it is for acute poisoning.

3. Chronic salicylism also leads to much more severe acidosis and has been associated with cases of marked fluid retention in the face of adequate intravascular fluid volume (SIADH).

B. Causes

1. The most common cause of chronic salicylism is administration of aspirin alone in too great of dose, especially in children under one year of age.

2. Another common cause of chronic aspirin poisoning is administration of multiple OTC medications which unknowingly (to the customer) also contain aspirin.

Vl. Prevention

A. Appropriate Use of Aspirin

1. The most severe instances of aspirin poisoning among infants and young children result from therapeutic overdosage. Nearly all cases involving young infants occur in this manner.

2. When aspirin is recommended, especially for a very young child, it is imperative that the parents not only be given very specific instructions as to the dosage and frequency of administration, but that they also be warned adequately as to the potential dangers of exceeding the recommended dose or of not ensuring an adequate fluid intake during the period of treatment.

3. Parents should always be informed when aspirin is being given in combination with other drugs so that they will not compound the effect by giving more aspirin to the feverish child on their own.

4. Parents should not use aspirin for young children without professional advice and approval. Parents feel compelled to give aspirin to their children upon the slightest provocation, and this should be discouraged. It is not always necessary that fever be combatted, and antipyretics are too often prescribed not really for the benefit of the child but rather for that of the physician or parents.

B. Safety Packaging

1. Voluntary limitation of the number of flavored children's (1 1/4 grain) aspirin tablets to 36 per bottle with a form of safety closure has had significant impact.

2. The Safety Packaging Act of 1970 should do much to prevent childhood poisonings in the future. Both effective safety closures and forms of unit packaging (which overtax the child's abilities and attention span and increase the likelihood of discovery before a toxic dose is ingested) are now available.

3. Parents must be cautioned to use closures properly and see that they are resecured.

(Adapted from Done, A.K. and Temple, A.R., "Treatment of Salicylate Poisoning," Mod. Treatment, 3:528-551 (Aug.) 1971).

V11. <u>Protocol for Management of Acute Salicylate Ingestion</u>

If the caller states that the child has ingested aspirin, the following steps should be undertaken:

1. Determine the amount that the child ingested and calculate the dose on a grain/lb or a mg/kg (preferred) basis.

(a) $$\frac{\text{no. pills taken} \times \text{mg ASA per pill}}{\text{weight of child in kg}} = \text{dose: mg/kg}$$

(b) $$\frac{\text{no. pills taken} \times \text{gr ASA per pill}}{\text{weight of child in lb}} = \text{dose: gr/lb}$$

Note: 1 grain = 65 mg
      1 kg = 2.2 lbs

2. If you can be sure that the child has ingested less than 1 gr/lb or less than 150 mg/kg no further therapy other than parental reassurance need be undertaken.

3. If the child has taken greater than 1 gr/lb or 150 mg/kg the child should have emesis induced immediately. This may be done at home and the child managed subsequently by parental observation, checking for increased respiratory rate or ringing in the ears.

4. If the child has ingested greater than 3.0 gr/lb or 400 mg/kg <u>or</u> if any symptoms of salicylate intoxication appear, the child should be evaluated by a physician in addition to immediate induction of emesis. The physician's evaluation should include:

a. determination of severity of symptoms of salicylate intoxication

b. evaluation of state of hydration

c. determination of serum salicylate level (minimum of 2, preferably 4 hours following ingestion)

5. Salicylate level should be compared to Done nomogram. If child fits the "moderate" or "severe" category of toxicity, he should be admitted for management. If the child fits the "asymptomatic" or "mild" category the child may be hydrated in the ER A second salicylate level should be obtained to evaluate the progression of the poisoning. Further action should be based on symptoms of the patient.

6. If hydration is to be accomplished in the emergency room, the amount of fluid given should be as follows:

   400 ml/M^2 given I.V. over 1 hr, using E-75 or Isolyte M (i.e., a fluid containing 40 mEq/l Na, 35 mEq/l K, 40 mEq/l Cl, and 20 mEq/l HCO_3).

7. If the child is admitted, the initial management step should be hydration, using something similar to the following:

   a. Initial hydration: 400 ml/M^2 over 1 hr, using a fluid containing 75 mEq/l Na, no K, 50 mEq/l Cl, and 25 mEq/l HCO_3.

   b. Subsequent fluid load: 2.5-3.5 l/M^2/24° of fluid containing 40 mEq/l Na, 35 mEq/l K, 40 mEq/l Cl, and 35 mEq/l HCO_3. (E 75, Isolyte M)

   c. If severe acidosis is present, an additional
      15 mEq/l NaHCO$_3$ should be added to the above
      solution.

8. Children with moderate to severe intoxication
   should be given 10 to 25 mg vitamin K prophy-
   lactically.

9. In "severe" intoxication, additional measures
   should be considered to increase the rate of
   removal of the salicylate. These may include:

   a. Osmotic diuresis using mannitol (but
      this only slightly increases the rate
      of removal).

   b. Alkalinization of the urine using sodium
      bicarbonate, THAM, or Diamox. (While
      this method is useful, it is difficult
      and produces additional complicating
      features to maintaining appropriate
      electrolyte balance.)

   c. Peritoneal dialysis with albumin contain-
      ing solution. (This is very effective--
      probably the most efficient procedure in
      small children.)

   d. Hemodialysis. (This is usually reserved
      for adults and is only rarely used.)

10. The most critical feature of the management of
    salicylate poisoning is good supportive measures.
    Careful monitoring of fluid and electrolyte
    parameters and other basic parameters, coupled
    with appropriate supportive care, is crucial.
    Such management is similar to the management
    of any illness.

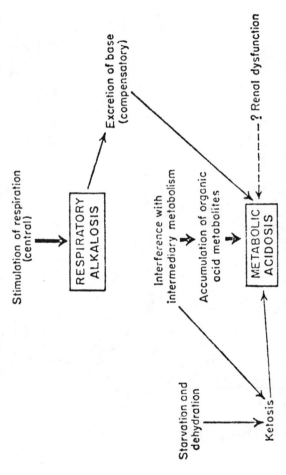

Figure 1.

Evolution of the acid-base disturbance in salicylate poisoning

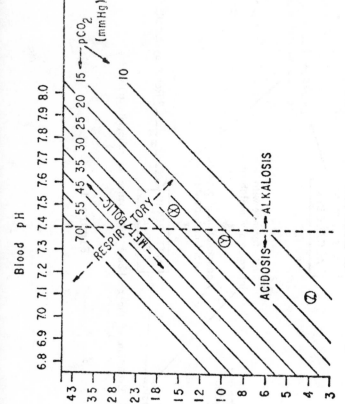

Figure 2.

Plot of blood pH and plasma CO_2 and pCO_2. Displacements produced as pure effects follow the "respiratory" or "metabolic" arrows; those between are results of either dual primary or compensatory secondary effects. "Normal" is at junction of "respiratory" and "metabolic" arrows (A). Typical disturbances of salicylate poisoning are shown: X = adult or older child with severe poisoning (partially compensated respiratory alkalosis); Y = infant with moderate, or older child with very severe, poisoning (mixed respiratory alkalosis and metabolic acidosis with normal to slightly acid pH); Z = infant with severe or prolonged poisoning (mixed disturbance, decompensated, with severe metabolic acidosis).

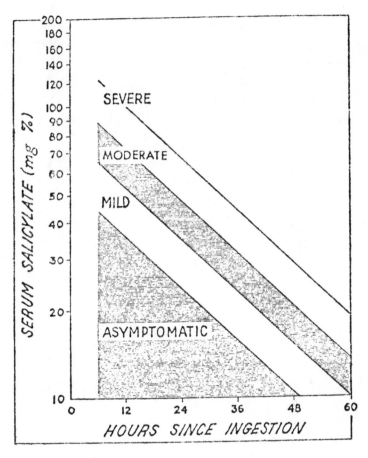

Nomogram for estimating the severity of poisoning from the serum salicylate level at varying intervals after ingestion of a single dose

Figure 3.

PESTICIDES AND SOLVENTS

Griffith E. Quinby, M.D., M.P.H., F.A.A.C.T.
Consultant, Clinical Toxicology, Wenatchee, Washington

PESTICIDE POISONING

The diagnosis of pesticide poisoning has long been
frought with error, false diagnosis, overemphasis,
and subterfuge by psychotics as well as malingerers (1).
While the practice of most specialties of medicine permit the clinician to rely upon the history given by
the patient, the friends, the family, employer or the
co-workers, there are a wide variety of reasons that
the initial presenting clinical history of pesticide
poisonings are incomplete, erroneous, or intentionally
misleading in the majority of cases. Unless the clinical toxicologist or his assistant re-investigate the
exposure history very, very thoroughly under conditions
assuming that each case history must be re-confirmed,
the wrong diagnosis and wrong management will take
place. This is particularly true of pesticide poisoning
cases reported to poison control centers, occupational
poisonings, public health reports, and news stories.
Within the last decade or so, scientists, politicians,
and even people without any valid qualifications in
environmental toxicology or ecology have frequently
overemphasized the risk-benefit ratio of pesticides
in efforts to eliminate or restrict manufacture and
use of certain pesticides. Use experiences have
definitely shown that certain pesticides should never
have gone on the market. The enactment of progressively restrictive laws has raised the requirements
of pre-registration experimental toxicology for the
introduction of new drugs and pesticides to the point
that it is no longer practical to apply common sense
to efforts to market new pesticide products or formulations unless the financial need for the new product
more than compensates for the astronomical cost of

pre-registration investigations. These considerations
have also beclouded the public's image of pesticides
adversely and have been good cause for incipient toxi-
phobic persons to become clinically active toxiphobes
whom any clinical toxicologist must expect to see in
his practice. Lesser overconcern with the real hazard
of pesticides is, of course, much more common and we
see these people more often in clinical toxicology
with their allegations of poisonings than we do bona
fide overt poisonings.

Our background index of suspicion that exposure
histories to pesticides are wrong or incomplete more
often than they are right should not be allowed to
keep us from reaching the proper deductive diagnosis
and instituting sometimes life-saving therapy when all
the presenting signs and symptoms fit the first facts.

Faced with a moribund patient or one rapidly approach-
ing this life-threatening situation, the clinical toxicologist is forced to use or commend his best clinical
judgment to institute specific therapy. This is especially critical in organic phosphorus poisoning when
supportive therapy is not the most modern available.
Therapy should be started even before laboratory tests
are ordered, much less drawn. This is the real dividing
line between the clinical toxicologist and the forensic
toxicologist or experimental toxicologist. The clinical toxicologist is primarily responsible for initial
therapy of poisoned patients. Other kinds of toxicologists should not be.

Suicide notes, workers' diagnoses, other patients'
impressions, and even general practitioners' clinical
impressions must be initially accepted as bona fide
evidence in health-threatening circumstances and therapy started on the basis of best toxicological impression while the clinical toxicologist or his co-workers
reinvestigate and reconfirm the exposure history as
originally presented. Sad to relate, general

practitioners have been too prone to accept too much
of their patients' impressions without confirmatory
re-investigation of the exposure history. What is
worse, the design of some state occupational health
insurance programs or laws will not pay the usual and
customary diagnostic costs if the diagnostician reaches
a differential diagnosis other than the presenting one.
This has lead many physicians and para-medical profes-
sions to accept without question the diagnoses as
originally alleged whether made by the worker, the
employer, or by others less qualified as diagnosticians.
Too many of our laws and regulations are based upon
such misinformation.

When the conditions of practices of a clinician pre-
clude or completely obviate his or her reinvestigation
of the exposure history, he should rely upon his next-
best representative or even public official such as
his technician, nurse, sanitarian, county agent, industrial hygienist, safety worker, research worker, and
like workers.

In his differential diagnosis, every clinical toxicologist should be prepared to recognize wrongly labelled
agents (2,3) or diagnosis of the first case, or epidemic
of a newly-recognized pesticide poisoning. With the
thousands of pesticide formulations already on the market
and more to come, we must expect to encounter new occupational disease syndromes, new ingestion-type poisonings,
and even new side effects of pesticides never published
before. In order to ensure optimal competence, you must
have available for easy reference a number of indexes
that identify brand, common and chemical names of pesticide products and related chemicals (4-8). If there
ever was a specialty in medicine that requires the
comprehension and utilization of chemical names, clinical toxicology is it! The clinical toxicologist who
attempts to rely upon proprietary names alone is invit-
ing a medical liability even greater than the general
practitioner who relies upon brand names of drugs alone

without knowing the common or chemical names of his
therapeutic agents.

Lest it be overlooked by some here, pesticides themselves sometimes do not account for the entire clinical
picture or are not nearly as hazardous as the vehicles,
solvents, impurities (9), adjuvants (pyrethrum), and
related chemicals that may be unintended ingredients
(10-15). The solvents of malathion cause death even
after the patient has recovered from ingesting malathion formulations.

For those of you about to become more active consult-
ing toxicologists, you must expect to recognize overtreatment and deaths resulting from overtreatment. Too
many inexperienced practitioners have reached wrong
diagnoses or have blindly followed rules of thumb in
therapy using antidotes such as atropine and pralidoxime.
I have unpublished case records of doctors using atropine
with and without pralidoxime long after the signs and
symptoms of pesticide poisoning were replaced by signs
and symptoms of poisoning by the two antidotes.

Clinical toxicologists are often consulted by private
lawyers and legal governmental authorities especially
the coroner's office to aid medical examiners in determining the cause of illness or death. The need for
thoroughness of case histories and examinations can not
be overemphasized. Laboratory studies should be planned
ahead as far as possible and when diagnosis is in doubt
save frequent blood samples and all body exudates separately for the first few passages and daily until a
fully sensible diagnosis can be made. It is much better
to waste some time collecting more samples than required
than to wish you had collected them to arrive at a proper
differential diagnosis. Autopsies should always be complete with special attention to cranial contents (which
is too often neglected). An EKG, EMG and electro enceph-
alogram must be considered in most thorough case studies.
Clinical neurologic and psychiatric exam should not be

overlooked in the proper diagnosis. Police and other field investigators' exposure histories must be rechecked for the frequent errors of judgment, such as a suicide being attributed to Captan just because the police brought in a bottle with a brand name of a soil fungicide that contained captan. Re-investigation revealed that the formulator had replaced the captan with dichlorethyl ether (16) without changing brand names at all.

Even the initial histories and clinical impressions of other toxicologists must be rechecked. A military pediatrician near Seattle with a great flair for toxicology of mushrooms, attributed a severe gastronenteritis and other symptoms to poisoning by Amanita phalloides without making careful inquiry into the characteristics (even the color) of the mushrooms ingested. Careful re-inquiry revealed that the two patients had eaten perfectly safe Morels but with them moldy ham and spoiled salmon containing heavy loads of food poisoning agents (17).

Whenever the signs and symptoms do not entirely fit the exposure history, even the chemical identity of the suspected toxicant must be verified. About 20 years ago a pesticide formulator accidentally bagged parathion in DDT bags resulting in many cattle deaths after they were dusted with the DDT bags (18). In a most recent case of polyneuritis in a spray painter reported at last year's meeting (19), the analysis of a common paint solvent in a gallon can revealed that someone at the plant had changed entirely the solvents in the can including one that could not easily be identified yet composing up to a third of the mixture.

SOLVENTS

There is some newer knowledge, unappreciated older knowledge, and deficiencies of knowledge of solvents that need inclusion in this paper.

One of the most important gaps in the physician's understanding of the clinical toxicology of solvents is that industrial solvents are to a degree crude mixtures of chemicals containing other chemicals either closely related structurally or greatly different in structure with toxic properties possibly far above or below the labelled or appreciated content. Part of the reason for inappreciation of this situation results from the confusing nomenclature of solvents.

While the field of pesticide chemistry has succinctly identified each active ingredient in mixtures designated by the idiom as "formulations" of vehicles, solvents, adjuvants, synergists, and impurities, the field of solvent chemistry either has not developed such a nomenclature or has not made it readily available to the physicians who need this identification of all ingredients in solvents. Moreover, there is frequent confusion of the general term "solvent". Too many people conceive solvents as containing only the single most active labelled ingredient and ignore the other ingredients. Too many people do not realize that many industrial solvents are mixtures of closely related or greatly different chemicals with purposely different solvency properties. Economics and the physics of production of solvents account for these different products. During the course of soliciting the speakers for the half-day symposium on solvents conducted at other times in this meeting, a great effort was made to find an industrial physician or chemist who would make a presentation on the manufacture, storage, transportation, distribution and sales up to the user or worker with solvents. No such speaker could be persuaded to cover these subjects. To my knowledge, no such presentation has ever been made before a toxicological meeting of any type. There is a great need for such a presentation as well as subsequent publication. No doubt the deficiency of such subject matter in the literature is due to the trade secrets as well as financial liabilities of the solvent producers and handlers being protected. It may be necessary to convince government regulatory bodies to require presentation of such a body of knowledge to prevent further unnecessary poisoning by unintended or unappreciated ingredients in solvents.

The recognition in 1975 that n-methyl butyl ketone (MBK) had caused epidemic polyneuropathy in cloth printers has pointed up the need for identifying those solvent formulations that contain MBK (20). Subsequent research has shown that MBK is synergized in experimental animals by methyl ethyl ketone MEK (21), and the occurrence of some cases in industry suggest that this may be true of man as well. The solvent n-hexane has long been known to cause polyneuropathy from use-experience (22), but only in the past year has there been a suggestion that 2-nitro propane may potentiate it and produce polyneuropathy at much lower acute exposure rate than was required by n-hexane alone.

Historically prior texts of clinical toxicology and other academic organizations did not identify clinical toxicology as a medical specialty. We are, in 1976, in our ninth year of formation of the American Academy of Clinical Toxicology, with a primary objective of identifying clinical toxicology as a separately recognized clinical specialty. Even though our American Board of Medical Toxicology is giving its second examination for certification, our Board is only in the preliminary stages of recognition by the American Board of Medical Specialties. We are now on the horizon of providing the very best and constantly improving diagnosis and treatment of poisoning that can be given not only to the people of North America but to all the world beyond. Workshops such as this are an excellent step in this direction and should be increased both in scope of content and the geographic areas served.

REFERENCES

1. Quinby GE: Management of intoxication from organophosphorus pesticides in aerial application. *AMA Congress on Occupational Health,* August, 1971.

2. Jackson TF, Halbert FL: A toxic syndrome associated with the feeding of polybrominated biphenyl-contaminated protein concentrate to dairy cattle. *JAVMA* 165:5:438-439, 1974.

3. Kolbye AC: Testimony at *Polybrominated Biphenyl Hearing,* Lansing, Michigan, May 29, 1975.

4. Frear DEH: *Pesticide Handbook-Entoma,* 1970.

5. Packer K (ed): *Farm Chemicals Magazine, Farm Chemical Handbook, 7 Sections (rev).* Meister Publishing, 1976.

6. *Nanogen Index: A Dictionary of Pesticides & Chemical Pollutants.* Nanogen International, 1975.

7. Billings SC, et al (eds): *Pesticide Handbook-Entoma, ed 26.* 1975-1976.

8. Thomson WT: *Agricultural Chemicals, Book I: Insecticides; Book II: Herbicides; Book III: Fumigants, Growth Regulators, Repellents, and Rodenticides; Book IV: Fungicides; (revised periodically).* Davis, California, 1970.

9. Milby TH, Epstein WL: Allergic contact sensitivity to malathion. *Arch Environ Hlth* 9:439, 1964.

10. Quinby GE: Physico-chemical changes in pesticides after formulation causing health hazards. *Soc of Toxicology,* Atlanta, Georgia, 1967.

11. Casida JE, Sanderson DM: Toxic hazards from

formulating the insecticide dimethoate in methyl 'cellosolve." *Nature* 189:507-508, 1961.

12. Fewkes FM, et al: Clay-catalyzed decomposition of insecticides. *Agri Food Chem* 8:203-210, 1960.

13. Lyman FL: Personal communications (with permission), from the Director of Industrial Medicine, Geigy Chemical Corporation, 1966.

14. Margot A, Gysin H: Diazinon: Its degradation products and their properties. *Helvetica Chimica Acta* 40:1562-1572, 1957.

15. Rosen, et al: The nature and toxicity of the photoconversion products of aldrin. *Bull Environ Contam & Tox*, in press.

16. Quinby GE: Coroner's misdiagnosis of cause of a suicidal ingestion: Captan vs dichlorethyl ether. Unpublished case report, 1963.

17. Quniby GE: Differential diagnosis of poisoning in consumers of morels. Case report presented before the Chelan Cty Medical Society, April, 1973.

18. Quinby GE, Cooper HR: An Epizootic of parathion Poisoning in Bulls Dusted with DDT-labelled Powder. Unpublished manuscript, 1955.

19. Quinby GE: Methyl n-butyl ketone solvent as a recently recognized cause of polyneuropathy. *Clin Tox* 8:363-364, 1975.

20. Allen N, et al: Solvent causes motor neuropathy at clothing factory. *JAMA* 229:247, 1974.

21. Spencer PS, et al: Nervous system degeneration produced by the industrial solvent methyl n-butyl ketone. *Arch Neurol* 32:219-222, 1975.

22.   Herskowitz A, et al: N-hexane neuropathy: A syndrome occurring as a result of industrial exposure. *New Engl J Med* 285:82, 1972.

PLANT AND MUSHROOM POISONING

K. F. Lampe, Ph.D.
Professor of Pharmacology and Anaesthesiology,
University of Miami School of Medicine

I. GENERAL CONSIDERATIONS

   A. To what extent is identification of the plant
      useful?

   B. Should the stomach be emptied in the absence
      of symptoms?

   C. Pediatric considerations.

II. CLASSES OF TOXIC PLANTS

   A. Gastroenteric Irritants

      a. Rapid onset: Plant ingestions producing a
         burning in the mouth, emesis, colic or diar-
         rhea shortly after ingestion (e.g., dieffen-
         bachia, wisteria, pokeweed) are managed
         symptomatically with particular attention to
         the prevention of dehydration. In the absence
         of systemic symptoms, serious complications
         are infrequent.

      b. Delayed onset: Plant ingestions associated
         with gastroenteritis appearing after a la-
         tent period of several hours or days are
         characteristic of toxalbumins. These toxins,
         found in the castor bean and rosary pea, are
         the most poisonous of plant origin. They
         inhibit protein systhesis which results in
         errosive disintegration of the entire diges-
         tive tract. Systemic involvement, when present,
         affects primarily the liver, spleen and kidney.

there is no specific therapy. Fluids,
electrolytes and a high glucose intake must
be provided.

B. Digitalis-Containing Plants

Initially there is local irritation to the mouth
followed by emesis. In contrast to the pure
cardiac glycosides, intoxications with oleander
or lily-of-the-valley will be associated with
colic and diarrhea due to the presence of sapo-
nins. Otherwise poisoning is similar to that
of digitalis overdosage which in a nor-kalemic
child with a healthy heart is usually characterized by conduction defects rather than increased
automaticity. The desirability of instituting
specific treatment should be based on the EKG.
First degree heart block requires only further
observation; with more advanced degrees of block
atropine may be employed. Disturbances in automaticity, in the absence of a conduction defect,
may be treated with oral potassium chloride.
Serious rhythm disturbances may require IV KCl
followed by oral medication for the following
several days. Intoxications exhibiting serious
involvement of the conduction system in conjunction with serious rhythm disturbances may
require the slow IV administration of diphenylhydantoin at 10 minute intervals (50-100 mg)
followed by additional 100 mg orally q6h for
the next several days.

C. Nicotine, Cystisine or Coniine Containing Plants

Ingestions of wild tobacco, laburnum seeds or
poison hemlock result in toxiocologically identical poisoning. Usually there is emesis within
15-60 minutes accompanied by a profuse salivation. Colic is minimal and diarrhea is unusual.
There may be headache, confusion, incoordination,

hyperpyrexia and sometimes mydriasis and tachycardia. Always administer charcoal as part of
therapeutic management. Respiratory support may
be required. Convulsions may occur and can be
suppressed if indicated.

D. Atropine Containing Plants

Such intoxications usually involve Jimson weed.
Atropine poisoning may be definitively diagnosed
in that it consistently produces equal bilateral
pupillary dilation, dry mouth and skin, loss of
bowel sounds and tachycardia. In severe cases
there may be pronounced elevation of body temperature and delirium. External cooling may be
indicated. Both the CNS and peripheral effects
can be antagonized by pysostigmine (pediatric
0.5 mg, adolescent 2 mg PRN).

E. Convulsion Producing Plants

Within 15-60 minutes of ingestion of one of the
water hemlocks, there will be a brief prodroma
of nausea, salivation, sometimes emesis and
tremors followed by one or more grand mal seizures. The treatment is as for status epilepticus.

III. CLASSES OF TOXIC MUSHROOMS

A. General Considerations

a. Variability of response.

b. Pediatric considerations.

c. Essential history taking in any mushroom
intoxication.

B. Toxic Mushrooms with a Rapid (under 2 hours)

Onset of Symptoms and Which are Rarely Associated with Fatalities

a. Gastroenteritis inducing

b. Hallucinogenic or deliriant

c. Sweat inducing

d. Alcohol sensitizing (Disulfiram like)

C. Toxic Mushrooms with a Delayed (over 6 hours) Onset of Symptoms and which have a Grave Prognosis Associated with Many Fatalities

a. Amanita phalloides-Type: The first sign of intoxication, usually occurring about 12 hours after ingestion, is a severe gastroenteritis with repeated emesis and a profuse, watery diarrhea. This usually clears in about 24 hours. There is then a brief, symptom-free interval which will be followed by progressive hepatic insufficiency (with or without jaundice), hypoglycemia, coagulation defects and coma. There may be a late appearing (3-5 days after ingestion) oliguria. The first phase of the intoxication is managed readily with fluid and electrolyte replacement. Therapy otherwise is identical to that for acute viral hepatitis with fulminant hepatic coma.

b. Gyromitra esculenta: The initial symptoms are fatigue, dizziness, headache and a feeling of fullness or abdominal pain. This is accompanied by intermittent emesis over the next several hours. In serious cases there is acute liver degeneration, usually associated with jaundice and progressive coma. Patients with an inherent glucos-6-phosphate dehydrogenase defficiency may experience massive erythrocyte hemolysis and consequent renal failure. The toxin is monomethylhydrazine and the treatment should be identical to that for an overdose of isoniazide, i.e., the daily IV administration of 100 mg pyridoxine and maintenance of a positive carbohydrate balance.

REFERENCES

1. Hardin JW, Arena JM: *Human Poisoning from Native and Cultivated Plants,* Duke University Press, 1974.

2. Kingsbury JM: *Poisonous Plants of the United States and Canada,* New York, Prentice Hall, 1964.

3. Lampe KF, Fagerstrom R: *Plant Toxicity and Dermatitis: A Manual for Physicians,* Williams & Wilkins, 1968.

SNAKES, SCORPIONS AND SPIDERS

Michael D. Ellis, M.S., R.Ph.
*Associate Director, University of Texas Medical Branch
Poison Center, Galveston, Texas*

SNAKES

The management of venomous snakebite is divided into
several schools of thought. The 3 primary management
regimens include: (a) initial incision of the wound,
followed by antivenin; (b) immediate debridement with
fasciotomy together with large doses of corticosteroids;
and (c) initial excision of the envenomated area with
removal of hemorrhagic tissue.

Initial incision and suction of the wound, if performed within 10-15 minutes of the envenomation can
remove up to 10% of the injected venom. After that
period of time the venom is bound to the tissue protein and suction is of little use. The use of antivenin has been the mainstay of treatment of venomous
snakebite. Although the antivenin specifically
neutralizes the injected Crotalidae venom, it will not
alter the extent of necrosis. Its equine origin also
makes the possibility of allergic manifestations considerable.

The administration of large doses of corticosteroids,
together with debridement and fasciotomy has been used
with some success, although appears to be somewhat
drastic for what is, at least initially, a relatively
local phenomenon.

Initial excision of the ecchymotic area and the
removal of the underlying hemorrhagic tissue physi-
cally removes the venom-containing tissue and thus
limits considerably the systemic symptoms and much of
the hematologic derangements which frequently occur.

In all three types of management strict attention must be paid to the volemic and hematologic status of the patient. Since all of the clotting factors are affected by the venom, upon arrival of the patient, a (a) Complete blood count, (b) Prothrombin time, (c) plasma fibrinogen level, (d) platelet count, and (d) partial prothrombin time should be obtained and repeated every 4-6 hours during the first 24 hours and daily thereafter.

SCORPIONS

There are about 40 plus species of scorpions found throughout the United States & Canada. Of these only 2 species are dangerously virulent to man, and these species are found almost exclusively in the state of Arizona and in Mexico.

The vast majority of scorpions, although usually producing an extremely painful, local area of swelling, that is sometimes accompanied by discoloration at the site of the sting, are not life-threatening, even to young children under normal conditions of health. Barring anaphylactic reactions, the sting requires little more than an ice pack. On the other hand, the stings of Centruroides sculpturatus and C. gertschi, the virulent Arizona scorpions, produce very little or no immediate local reaction. Their venom is extremely neurotoxic and deaths have resulted.

SPIDERS

Nearly all spiders have the ability to bite. For the most part these wounds respond to local treatment. The bite of the black widow spider and the brown recluse or fiddle-back spider are considerably more serious.

The black widow has classical markings, making her hard to misidentify. The bitten area may or may not

show two tiny red spots where the spider's fangs pene-
trated. Initially there is local pain, lasting 1-2
hours. Depending on the area bitten, next follows
local muscle cramping. The pain characteristically
spreads to the abdomen where the muscles assume a
board-like rigidity. Antivenin is available for
counteracting the effects of the injected venom.

The brown recluse or fiddle-back spider is the other
spider that causes major medical problems. The bite
of this spider usually goes unnoticed, as no pain is
associated with it. This is followed by a red, swollen,
tender area that breaks down leaving a draining, sharply
demarcated ulcer with a base of granulation tissue.
The ulcer can vary in size from a few millimeters to
3-4 cm. and total excision of the wound followed by
grafting if necessary, is frequently required.

TOXICITY OF SOAPS, DETERGENTS AND CAUSTICS

Anthony R. Temple, M.D.
Director, Intermountain Regional Poison Control Center
Associate Professor of Pediatrics, University of Utah
  College of Medicine
Associate Professor of Clinical Pharmacology and
  Toxicology, University of Utah, College of Pharmacy

Joseph C. Veltri, B.S., R.Ph.
Associate Director, Intermountain Regional Poison
  Control Center and Drug Information Service, Salt
  Lake City

I. Epidemiology and Availability

Of the estimated one to two million poisonings annually in the United States, approximately half of these involve household products, of which soaps, detergents, and caustics make up a significant portion. There were 21,243 exposures to soaps, detergents, and caustics reported to the National Clearinghouse for Poison Control Centers in 1972.

From a toxicologic perspective, these products are of considerable importance, because:

   a. Product ingredients may be irritating to
      human tissues.
   b. Functionally, they are high use products.
   c. They are stored in the home in areas of con-
      venient access, often in areas accessible to
      children.

Soaps are a class of agents frequently used in the home for personal hygiene. They have generally been replaced by other agents for laundry use since minerals in hard water react with soap to form insoluble substances called scum. Scum tends to settle on clothes and give them a gray color. When soaps are used to launder clothes, manufacturers often used "builders" in the soap to maintain alkalinity in the wash water. Builders are usually inorganic salts (usually mildly alkaline phosphates) that promote wetting and emulsification. Light duty soaps are unbuilt; heavy duty soaps contain builders. Soap are composed entirely of the salts (Na/K) of fatty acids.

Detergents are made from petroleum and from natural fats and oils. They include such compounds as Na, K. and NH_3 salts of fatty acids, sulfonated hydrocarbons, and phosphorylated hydrocarbons. The chemical processes that produce detergents are more complex than the reaction between fat and lye that makes soap. The properties of detergents depend on their chemical composition. Because a greater diversity of raw materials and chemical processes is used in making detergents than in making soaps more types of detergents are available.

Detergents dissolve readily in water, hot or cold, soft or hard. They do not form scum in hard water. Some make suds easily, others clean with little or no suds. Like soaps, packaged detergents come in two types--light duty (unbuilt) and heavy duty (built), and in liquid, powdered, and tablet forms.

Before July, 1965, some surfactants widely used in household detergents decomposed very slowly in sewage treatment plants or surfact waters. The low rate of degradation of these "hard" (high phosphate) detergents, plus their tendency to foam at very low concentrations, was a major factor in the much-publicized foam problem. Another disadvantage of phosphates is that they may contribute to the growth of algae. Household detergent now on the market contain surfactants that are more readily decomposed by microrganisms during treatment of sewage. As a result, less detergent gets into streams to cause foam. Such detergents are called biodegradable or low phosphates. Decreasing the phosphate content requires increasing the alkalinity of most detergents making them more irritating to tissue.

Common strong acids include sulfuric, hydrochloric, nitric, perchloric, pally sodium hydroxide, or potassium hydroxide. The most common agents involved in pediatric exposures are liquid and crystalline drain cleaners, oven cleaners, toilet bowl cleaners and ammonia.

II. PRODUCT CHARACTERISTICS

A. Definitions

Soap - a salt of fatty acid, usually made by the action of alkali on natural fats and oils or on the fatty acids obtained from fat or vegetable oils. The major use is for cleaning, particularly skin.

Detergent - non-soap surfactants in combination with inorganic ingredients, generally in the form of phosphates, silicates, and carbonates. The major uses are for cleansing clothing or other household items to ensure a bright, non-scum effect.

Caustic - agents generally strong alkalis or acids, which produce severe tissue destruction following topical contact. The major uses are for heavy duty cleaning of surfaces.

Builder - extra alkaline salts, such as phosphates, silicates, or carbonates, which are added to soaps to help soften the water and facilitate the removal of certain types of soils.

Enzyme - proteolytic enzymes used to remove otherwise difficult stains (e.g., blood, grass, and some foods), which are incorporated into some laundry detergents or laundry soaps.

B. Chemical Classification

1. Soap
2. Synthetic detergents
   a. anionic surfactants
   b. nonionic surfactants
   c. cationic surfactants
   d. phosphates
   e. silicates
   f. carbonates
3. Sodium hypochlorite, peroxide, or perborate
4. Ammonia
5. Caustics
   a. acids (sulfuric, nitric, hydrochloric, etc.)
   b. alkalis (sodium hydroxide, potassium hydroxide)

C. Product Classification

Products can be classified as:
1. Regular soaps
2. Synthetic detergents
   a. light duty products
   b. heavy duty (general purpose of laundry) products
   c. enzyme pre-soak products
   d. hard surface cleaners
   e. automatic dishwashing detergents
   f. scouring cleansers
3. Ammonia, drain cleaners, bleaches
   a. household and industrial ammonia
   b. chlorine bleaches
   c. caustic drain cleaners

III. TOXICOLOGY

A. Modes of Toxicity

The usual modes through which toxic effect are produced are:

1. Skin exposure
2. Eye instillation
3. Ingestion

B. Toxicology of Individual Product Categories

1. Soaps

The toxicity of soaps is generally quite low.
Since fatty acids are mild irritants, exposure
to soaps may product cutaneous, ocular, oral
or gastrointestinal irritation. Ingestion of
large amounts of soap may induce emesis or
produce mild diarrhea.

2. Detergents

Detergents are generally of low toxicity,
except in those cases where the formulations
result in a relatively high degree of alkalinity.

a. Non-ionic surfactants - These agents are
medium to long-chain sulfonates and include
alkyl arly polyether sulfates, alcohols or
sulfonates. They are common to low-sudsing
detergents. Their toxicity is quite low,
but can produce mild cutaneous, ocular,
oral or gastrointestinal irritation. Ingestion of large amounts may induce emesis
or produce a milk diarrhea.

b. Anionic surfactants - These agents are
salts of fatty acids, sulfonated hydrocarbons, and phosphorylated hydrocarbons,
one of the most common being the alkyl-
benzenesulfonates. They are common to
general laundry detergents. By themselves,
their toxicity is low, causing local irritation to skin, eye, oral or gastrointestinal mucosa. Ingestions may result in

emesis or mild diarrhea. The addition
of builders to detergents plays a significant role in the product's actual toxicity.
The phosphates, and in particular, sodium
tripolyphosphate, add only slightly to the
general irritant and emetic quality of the
detergent. However, the use of silicates
and carbonates as in "low phosphate" detergents, or certain phosphates such as
trisodium phosphates, may raise the alkalinity of the product and increase significantly its irritant quality. Highly
alkaline detergent products may produce
severe ocular irritation, oral burns,
esophageal burns, and bloody gastritis.
Certain electric dishwashing detergents
typify those agents with a much higher
degree of alkalinity and many of these
products should be considered to have toxic
effects similar to caustics. In general,
the toxicity of liquid detergents is lower
than that of the powders or granules, because of their formulations in aqueous or
hyroalcoholic solutions. Additives to detergents, such as bleaches, enzymes or
bacteriocidal agents, are usually in low
concentrations and do not influence the
overall product toxicity.

c. Cationic surfactants - These agents are
quaternary ammonium compounds, such as
benzalkonium chloride, benzethonium chloride, and cetylpyridinium chloride, and
substituted alkyl quaternary compounds
like dimethyl disterayl ammonium chloride.
They are frequently used as disinfectants
and found in fabric softeners. Cationic
detergents are much more toxic than anionic
or nonionic detergents, with the double
side-chain substituted compounds being

less toxic than the single side-chain
substituted ones. Concentrated solutions
have caustic qualities, while more dilute
solutions have marked irritant effects.
In addition to these local or topical effects,
systemic absorption also produces toxic symptoms, including CNS effects, such as a feeling of apprehension, restlessness, confusion,
convulsions, respiratory paralysis, muscle
weakness, and cyanosis.

3. Bleaches

These agents contain varying concentrations
of sodium peroxide, sodium perborate, or
sodium hypochlorite. The most commonly used
household bleaches contain approximately 3-6%
solutions of sodium hypochlorite in water.
Granular bleaches have higher concentrations
of agents and are therefore more toxic. Commercial bleaches contain peroxides or perbor-
ates and are of such concentration that they
can be similar to caustics in their toxicity.
Household bleaches, however, are mild irritants
and have only rarely been associated with any
degree of tissue destruction. They result in
skin or eye irritation, mild oral or esophageal
burns, or gastrointestinal irritation. They
may produce emesis in higher concentrations.
As indicated, other bleaches may produce much
more severe irritation and should be treated
accordingly.

As a note of interest, mixing hypochlorites
with other household cleaning agents can result in the release of gases which are irritating to the pulmonary tract and may result in
pulmonary edema if the exposure is severe
enough. The following are the most typical
reactions:

    a. Hypochlorites mixed with strong acids releases chlorine gas.

    b. Hypochlorite mixed with ammonia releases chloramine gas.

4. Ammonias

As with bleaches, most household ammonias contain weak solutions of ammonia. Industrial ammonias may be much more concentrated. Weak ammonia solutions are mild irritants. Very concentrated solutions may be caustic.

5. Caustics

While both alkalis and acids can cause tissue destruction, there is a difference. Acids produce a coagulation necrosis which tends to cause a superficial type of damage, rather deep, penetrating type of burn. Alkalis tend to cause a necrosis which is deep and penetrating, often resulting in severe effects such as esophageal perforation. These more deep burns are associated with much more severe scarring and stricture formation. These agents combine with protein to form proteinates and with fats to form soap, thus producing penetrating burns on contact with tissue. Toxicity is related to causticity. Damage is related to concentration of the agent and length of time that it's in contact with the tissue.

    a. Skin exposures

Spills of caustics onto the skin may produce first or second degree, and, occasionally, third degree burns depending on concentration and duration of contact.

b. Eye exposures

Spills of caustics into the eye can cause
a variety of effects. In the mild exposure,
the conjunctiva and cornea may be infected
and mildly edematous. In more severe cases,
intraocular damage is seen, corneal erosions
occur and subsequent scarring, perforation,
and blindness may occur.

c. Ingestions

After ingestion, burns usually appear about
the lips, on the face, and in the oropharynx.
If the product is swallowed, burns of the
hypopharynx, epiglottis and esophagus may
occur. Burns of the esophagus may occur
even if there are no burns noted in the
mouth. Burns of the esophagus may result
in performation and mediastinitis or may
result in subsequent scarring and stricture
formation.

Following the initial insult, a number of
ensuing complications may arise. Aspiration
pneumonitis, mediastinitis, glottic edema,
or shock may all contribute significant
morbidity and may result in death.

When burns are not accompanied by acute
complications, the pain and difficulty
swallowing will abate within a few days,
after which there is a period during which
the patient is relatively free of symptoms.
During this period strictures may develop,
which result in dysphagia and weight loss.
The most severe strictures occur in circum-
ferential burns. While most of these
strictures are in the esophagus, ingestions
of acids may result in pyloric strictures
in the stomach.

IV. <u>MANAGEMENT</u>

   A. <u>Emergency Management</u>

      1. In all cases of ingestions involving soaps, detergents, or caustics, immediate dilution with water or milk should be instituted. In cases where irritation is anticipated demulcent therapy should be instituted.

      2. In all cases of eye instillation or skin exposure, immediate irrigation using water or an ophthalmic irrigating solution should be instituted and continued for 10-15 minutes.

      3. Ensure an adequate airway. Consider endotracheal intubation or tracheotomy if acute respiratory obstruction occurs following glottic burns.

      4. Emesis should not be induced nor should gastric tubes be placed.

   B. <u>Patient Evaluation</u>

      1. Thorough examination of all exposed surfaces, with particular attention given to the oropharynx should be made.

      2. With caustics, even when there are no visible burns in the oropharynx, burns in the esophagus are possible. When there are burns in the mouth, there may not be burns in the esophagus. Therefore, all patients should have esophagoscopy performed.

      3. A chest x-ray should be obtained in all patients with respiratory symptoms.

C. Management of Burns

1. Burns of the skin, eye, and oropharynx may require analgesics for pain.

2. Burns of the esophagus may result in pain on swallowing or esophageal-gastric spasm. Therefore, giving a liquid diet or making the patient N.P.O. is indicated for 48-72 hours.

3. The use of cortiocosteroids is controversial. Although some uncontrolled studies have reported that steroids did not prevent edema or esophageal stricture, many experienced clinicians favor their use beginning immediately after injury and continuing in higher dosage for several weeks. The appropriate daily dose of corticosteroids is prednisone 1-2 mg/kg or its equivalent.

4. If tissue injury is seen or is suspected, some clinicians favor antimicrobial prophylaxis. Most, however, believe that prophylactic antibiotics will promote superinfection by resistant bacteria and fungi and should not be used. Animal studies suggest that if steroids are used, they should be given concommitantly with antibiotics.

D. Management of Complications

1. Pneumonitis or mediastinitis should be treated with adequate and appropriate antibiotics following culture proven infections.

2. Strictures need surgical intervention, bougenage, surgical repair or colonic interposition.

V. <u>PROGNOSIS</u>

A. <u>Soaps and Detergents</u>

While the toxic effects may be temporarily painful or discomforting, the effects are generally
reversible and no permanent damage occurs.

B. <u>Caustics</u>

1. One-third of all oral "ingestions" will result in esophageal burns.
2. Ten to fifteen percent of victims with
esophageal burns will develop strictures.
3. Of those with severe esophageal burns some
may die from immediate effects and others
may have irreversible damage done. The
prognosis is not pleasant.

VI. <u>SUMMARY</u>

In spite of the fact that eye exposures and oral
ingestions of soaps and detergents are a frequent problem,
the irritant effects caused by them are short-lived and
reversible. The same appears to be true with the usual
household concentrations of ammonia and bleaches, but
this is not universally the case, and to be safe, severe
irritation (first-degree burns) should be anticipated.
On the other hand, caustics produce severe burns
(second and third-degree) leading to permanent eye
damage, esophageal or gastric perforation or strictures.
Caustics must be evaluated and treated vigorously.
Oral ingestions should be evaluated with esophagoscopy
whenever possible. Careful therapy and follow-up is a
must following caustic exposures.

ETHANOL INTOXICATION

Helmut M. Redetzki, M.D.
Professor and Head, Department of Pharmacology and Therapeutics, Louisiana State University School of Medicine, Shreveport, Louisiana

ABSTRACT

Alcohol intoxication either in its pure form or complicated by concomitanting ingestion of drugs affecting the central nervous system, is one of the most common toxicological syndromes encountered in hospital emergency rooms and other medical treatment facilities. With accidental, intentional or suicidal ingestions of alcohol, age of patients ranges from infancy to senescence. Sources for the ingested alcohol vary widely including the various forms of beverages as well as mouthwashes, cosmetics, elixirs, solvents and denatured alcohol.

PHARMACOLOGY

Ethanol is a central nervous system depressant that causes stupor, coma and eventually death if ingested in excessive quantities. With prolonged drinking sprees, cumulation of congeners (methanol, ethyl acetate, as well as higher straight-and branched-chain alcohols) may contribute to the manifestations of toxicity and hangover.

Alcohol is most efficiently and rapidly absorbed from the small intestine, where the large mucosal surface area aides diffusion. Absorption from the stomach is delayed by food or high concentration of consumed alcohol. Peak blood levels after single rapid ingestion or cessation of protracted drinking are reached within 30 minutes to 3 hours.

Alcohol is readily distributed in the body according
to the water space. It is metabolized in the liver
mainly by alcohol dehydrogenase. The physiological
role of the microsomal ethanol oxidizing system
(MEOS) is still open to discussion. Elimination of
ethanol by kidneys and lungs is of minor significance
ranging from approximately 2% of total ingested alcohol (with low dosages) to 10% (with high dosages).
The rate of alcohol oxidation expressed as decline
of blood alcohol concentration per hour varies from
10 mg/100 ml hour to 35 mg/100 ml/hour (average 15
mg/100 ml/hour). Blood alcohol curves do not always
follow straight line (0 order) function. Shock and
emesis can lead to alterations in circulating blood
volume which may temporarily reduce the rate of
decline.

RANGE OF TOXICITY

Each ounce of whiskey, glass of wine or bottle of
beer (12 ounces) can raise blood alcohol level by
about 25 mg%. The term "proof" expresses double the
alcohol concentration in volume %. Rule of thumb
is that one ml/kg of absolute ethanol results in
blood levels of 100 mg% two hours after ingestion.
Lethal dose for adults is 5 g/kg to 8 g/kg of body
weight, that for children approximately 3 g/kg.

CLINICAL EFFECTS

Blood levels below 50 mg% rarely lead to marked
sensory or motor impairment. Values above 150 mg%
are consistent with intoxication as manifested by
staggering gait, nausea and vomiting. Lethal blood
alcohol values can range from 350 mg% to 700 mg%,
alcoholics usually tolerating higher levels than
abstainer, children less than adults. Lethal levels
may be substantially lower when alcohol has been
ingested together with sedatives, hypnotics or
tranquilizers. Hypoglycemia eventually terminating

in convulsions is a serious complication of acute
alcoholic intoxication especially in children and
skid row alcoholics (glycogen depleted liver with
impaired gluconeogenesis). Some cases show moderate
metabolic acidosis (lactacidemia), few progress to
frank ketoacidosis with markedly increased β hydro-
xybutyrate levels (enhanced release of free fatty
acids from adipose tissue). Peripheral vasodilation
and central nervous system depression lead to hypothermia. Skin may initially appear flushed but later
becomes cold and clammy with grayish cyanosis. Deep
tendon reflexes may disappear. Death is usually
caused by respiratory failure, rarely by cardiac
dysfunction and shock.

ASSESSMENT OF THE INTOXICATED PATIENT

Check vital signs, monitor heart rate and blood
pressure. Obtain arterial blood gases, blood glucose,
BUN and electrolytes. Get blood alcoholic determination and urine screen or coma panel. Check for
occult bleeding, obtain blood count and hematocrit.
Check for head injury (skull film and lumbar puncture).
The chronic alcoholic is susceptible to pulmonary
infections (impaired defense system, gastric aspirations) but may show little increase in temperature or
white cell count.

Since blood alcohol determinations are time consuming and might not be available on a stat basis,
we recommend that in all serious cases blood is
immediately analyzed for serum (or plasma) osmolality.
A blood alcohol concentration of 100 mg% increases
osmolality by approximately 28-30 milliosmoles/kgH$_2$0.
If osmolality is normal or only slightly increased,
alcohol intoxication can be excluded as cause of coma.
Search for subdural hematoma, evidence of stroke
or drug overdose. Alcohol might only be incidentally,
but not causally, related to unconsciousness (odor of
breath can be misleading). A high serum osmolality

confirms diagnosis and gives good approximation of blood level (exclude hypernatremia, diabetic coma and uremia by checking Na, glucose and BUN values).

TREATMENT

Patients with mild or moderate intoxication do not need special treatment; but should be kept under observation. The severely intoxicated patient is at risk and is best treated in a detoxification unit. The patient in alcoholic coma represents a medical emergency and should be treated in the medical intensive care unit.

The following recommendations apply to the severely intoxicated or comatose patient.

1. Check respiration (normal tidal volume is approximately 10-15 cc/kg). If necessary, establish airway and provide respiratory support.

2. Place patient in semi-lateral decubitus position with head forward and mouth down to avoid aspiration of vomitus.

3. Assess fluid needs, start iv drip. Chronic alcoholics are often fluid overloaded; however, patients with protracted vomiting may have substantial fluid deficits.

4. Induction of emesis is rarely indicated. Gastric lavage can be helpful if large amounts of alcohol have been ingested within one to two hours or if concurrent ingestion of other dangerous drugs is known or suspected. Intubation with a cuffed endotracheal tube is needed to protect the depressed or comatose patient. Insertion of a levine tube with continuous aspiration of gastric secretions is often beneficial.

5. Suspect alcoholic hypoglycemia in any case with unusual neurological findings, convulsions or coma. Administer 50-100 ml of 50% glucose iv if blood glucose is below 60 mg% or if lab data are not available. Always combine this with im injection of 100 mg thiamine. Continue with iv drip of D5W.

6. Moderate metabolic acidosis (identifiable through anion gap or blood gas analysis) is usually sufficiently controlled by fluid therapy. Use bicarbonate only with severe acid-base derangements.

7. Hemodialysis can eliminate alcohol 3-4 times more rapidly than liver metabolism. It may be useful in patients with excessive blood levels, impaired hepatic function and in those whose condition deteriorates in spite of standard treatment.

STATUS OF FRUCTOSE AS AN ACCELERATOR OF ETHANOL METABOLISM

In spite of continuing publications and studies indicating that fructose accelerates the rate of alcohol metabolism, these claims are challenged by numerous investigators. We do not recommend use of fructose either by the oral or parenteral route. The modest (if any) reduction in the duration of intoxication period is outweighed by a variety of side effects which range from upper abdominal and retrosternal pain, apprehension, itching and burning of skin to nausea, vomiting and shock. It has also been established that fructose can intensify an existing metabolic acidosis, deplete the liver of adenine nucleotides and dehydrate patients through its osmotic diuretic effect. Utilization of fructose is probably contraindicated for patients with advanced liver disease, uncontrolled diabetes mellitus, shock, hyperuricemia and hypoxic states.

ALCOHOL WITHDRAWAL

With gradual decline of blood alcohol levels the
chronic alcoholic enters the first phase of withdrawal
which is characterized by anxiety, tremors and hyper-
acuity of sensory modalities. In most patients
hyperventilation with moderate respiratory alkalosis
can be detected. Magnesium values often decline
temporarily and the patient may suffer convulsions.
They occur early in the withdrawal phase (first to
third day), are usually not severe and rarely need
intensive therapy. Withdrawal from chronic alcohol
abuse can be ameliorated by oral or parenteral administration of benzodiazepines (chlordiazepoxide
or diazepam are used frequently). Phenytoin 300 to
400 mg/day seems to offer additional protection
against alcohol induced withdrawal seizures. Treatment of the delirium phase is demanding. It requires
general supportive measures, replacement of fluids
and electrolytes, sedation (benzodiazepines,
paraldehyde). Phenothiazines (chlorpromazine or
mesoridazine) lack sufficient cross-tolerance to
substitute for alcohol but are very effective in the
treatment of abnormal excitement occuring during the
early detoxification phase.

REFERENCES

1. Amene PC: Intravenous fructose for acute alcoholism: A double blind study. *JACEP*
   5:253-256, 1976.

2. Bueno F, Mezey E: Management of alcoholism.
   Rat Drug Ther 10:1-8, 1976.

3. Cooperman MT, Daivdoff F, Spark R, Pallotta J:
   Clinical studies of alcoholic ketoacidosis.
   Diabetes 23:433-439, 1974.

4. Jacob MS, Sellers EM: Emergency management of
   alcohol withdrawal. *Drug Ther* 2:28-34, 1977.

5. Kekomaki M, Raivio KO, Maenpaa PH: Interference
   with liver metabolism by d-fructose. *Acta Anesth
   Scand Supp* 37:114-118, 1970.

6. Levy LJ, Duga J, Girgis M, Gordon EE: Ketoacidosis
   associated with alcoholism in nondiabetic subjects. *Ann Int Med* 78:213-219, 1973.

7. Redetzki HM, Koerner TA, Hughes JR, Smith AG:
   Osmometry in the evaluation of alcohol intoxication. *Clin Tox* 5:343-363, 1972.

8. Seixas FA: Alcohol and its drug interactions.
   Ann Int Med 83:86-92, 1975.

9. Sellers EM, Kalant H: Alcohol intoxication and
   withdrawal. *New Eng J Med* 294:757-762, 1976.

10. Walden AI, Redding JS, Faillace L, Steenburg E:
    Rapid detoxification of the acute alcoholic with
    hemodialysis. *Surgery* 66:201-207, 1969.